IBS
GUT INSTINCT

The Definitive Solution For Improving Gut Health

Treating Irritable Bowel Syndrome And Attaining Gut Bliss

Larry Siebert Ph.D.

Visit us at

http://www.LarrySiebert.com

Or

For mp3s visit our sister site at

http://www.HypnoCDStore.com

DISCLAIMER

The information in this book is not a substitute for the medical advice and recommendations of physicians or other licensed health care providers. The information in this book is for informational educational purposes, and is intended to help the reader cooperate with physicians and health professionals to improve their health. This book is not attempting to prescribe any medical treatment, since under the laws of the United States, only a licensed healthcare provider can do so. The reader should regularly consult a physician in matters relating to their health and particularly with respect to any symptoms that may require diagnosis or medical attention.

The publisher and the author are not responsible for any products or services offered or referred to in this book and expressly disclaim all liability in connection with the use of any such products or services and for any damage, loss, or expense to person or property arising out of or relating to them.

All names and identifying details contained in this book have been changed to protect the privacy of those individuals.

TABLE OF CONTENTS

CHAPTER

TABLE OF CONTENTS

CHAPTER

INTRODUCTION

IF I CAN SHOW YOU HOW TO REDUCE OR ELIMINATE YOUR IBS SYMPTOMS, WOULD YOU BE INTERESTED IN LEARNING MORE?

I'm about to reveal a method that can assist you in finally overcoming your IBS symptoms, and here's the best part:

THERE ARE NO SUPPLEMENTS TO TAKE, THERE IS NO CHANGE TO YOUR DIET AND THERE IS NO USE OF MEDICATION REQUIRED!

I know that's a bold statement, but I can confidently say that because I've been personally using this approach with clients for over a decade. And trust me when I say **IT WORKS**. If my word is not proof enough for you, then you'll find that this book contains medical references from over thirty years of study that agree with me.

THIS METHOD IS 3X MORE EFFECTIVE THAN STANDARD MEDICAL TREATMENT!

Standard medical treatment for IBS (which changes what you eat and gives you medication) has not been able to satisfactorily improve or lessen IBS symptoms; in fact, it's only effective for 25% of the population. To date there is no known single cause for IBS and medical science has no single effective treatment either.

In "*IBS Gut Instinct*," you will learn about a specific technique that will help you overcome your IBS symptoms. While almost all other books about IBS tell you what foods to eat and what foods not to eat, they don't tell you that **FOODS ARE NOT THE SOURCE** of the problem.

This method is clinically proven, and yes, it has helped people just like you reduce or eliminate their IBS symptoms; and the fact is that studies show this method is effective 70% to 90% of the time. If you are one of these people, I promise you that you will get your life back.

My name is Dr. Larry Siebert and my Doctoral degree is in Clinical Hypnotherapy. I've been in private practice in the San Francisco Bay Area since 1996, and have traveled thousands of miles to attend trainings in the area of personal growth. Many of those trainings have been in the area of how the mind and body communicate to promote emotional and physical healing.

It's this communication that we'll be using. Why will we be using mind-body communication? Because it has been proven effective in reducing or eliminating IBS symptoms, that's why.

HERE IS A PREVIEW OF WHAT YOU'LL LEARN ...

- What's Different About This Book On IBS
- What Causes IBS
- How Is IBS Diagnosed, and What The Guidelines Are
- Current Strategies For Treating IBS

- Can Changes In Diet Reduce IBS Symptoms

- How Good Is Pharmacological Treatment

- Is It Possible To Use Imagery In Healing

- How Mind-Body Communication Affects Your IBS Symptoms

- The Case for Using Gut-Directed Hypnotherapy

- And Much, Much More!

IT'S TIME TO
TAKE CONTROL
OF YOUR LIFE TODAY

Are you or a loved one suffering from IBS? If you're ready to take your life back from all the problems related to IBS, then this is the book for you.

Don't wait to get the information you need to return to an active and fulfilling life. If you're ready to learn about this highly effective method, a method that will keep you active, a method that will have you enjoying life again, then it's time to take action today.

I know that living with IBS can be stressful, so let's move on the next chapter and I'll see if I can help a little with that.

WANT THE
BONUS RECORDING?

DID I MENTION IT'S FREE?

I wanted to give you a little bonus to immediately help you with your IBS symptoms. This bonus recording is called 10 Minutes to Relaxation. It is an mp3 file that can be downloaded right now.

This audio recording is similar to the recordings that I use when working with patients, except that this recording does NOT contain any brainwave entrainment. This recording is meant to reduce stress and relax you in 10 minutes. You may already be aware that stress causes your IBS symptoms to worsen, so listening to this recording will help reduce your stress and therefore reduce your IBS symptoms.

I know some of you are asking, "How do I get this bonus information?" Well it's really easy. All you need to do is to go to the website page I setup:

http://www.LarrySiebert.com/ibsgi

You'll see a picture of the book cover so you'll know that you're on the correct page. You'll also see a large down arrow pointing you to fill in your name and your email address. After that all you need to do is click on "Instant Access." Within a couple of minutes you'll receive an email that contains a link to the 10 Minute to Relaxation file.

I'll repeat this later on:

**Never listen to hypnotic recordings
while driving a car or operating machinery**

When listening to hypnosis recordings choose an environment that is quiet and safe. Using headphones typically will reduce outside noise; however this is not necessary to become relaxed.

Save the link to your computer, enjoy the recording, and then go to the next chapter and read what's different about this IBS book.

3

WHAT'S DIFFERENT ABOUT THIS BOOK ON IBS?

If you are like most people that are reading this book, then you've probably had IBS for over one year under your doctor's supervision without much relief. Of course you could have recently been diagnosed with IBS also and are just trying to find a solution. In either case, your doctor probably had you make changes to your diet, and possibly prescribed some type of medication. Since your doctor made changes to your diet, if you're like most IBS sufferers, you have investigated and read many types of books about diets. In fact, most books that are written about Irritable Bowel Syndrome (IBS) are about diet.

Following your doctor's recommendations, most IBS sufferers like yourself have become an expert on what to eat and of course what not to eat. I'm sure that you have read the IBS cookbooks with recipes for breakfast, lunch, and dinner, and not surprisingly these recipes are supposed to be great tasting, right? To become an expert on the foods related to your condition, you've probably read books that contain fiber charts, and whole-food recipes, as well as books related to low-starch diets, no starch diets, low-carb diets, and natural eating diet plans.

I know that there are also books available on IBS that have ancient cures, easy cures, fast cures, simple cures, and super food cures. Of course there are even new solutions, science-based solutions, clinically-proven solutions, and not surprisingly the ultimate solution. There are books on reducing pain through diet as well as pain-free strategies. You can even use probiotics to balance your gut. There is the gluten connection and the lactose connection and the gut bacterial connection. There are even books to control your IBS in one week! And if that actually worked there would be no more books written on solving IBS problems. And sure enough I'm sure you have come across the natural-cure books.

If after you've tried all of the above type of books without success, then you might have turned to the books that tell you how to take control and conquer your IBS. Or maybe you've even looked into books that talk about managing your IBS, and there are still other books that tell you what to do when it flares up. There are step-by-step methods; some are six steps, or seven steps, or even ten steps. Some books are about what to do when you're first diagnosed with IBS.

If still none of these books are working for you, then it's natural to start reading books that are titled, "What your doctor doesn't know about IBS," because these changes to your diet and the medication that your doctor might be prescribing simply is not working well enough for you.

Do you know why there are so many books written about IBS and diet? In all likelihood it's because conventional medical treatment for IBS mainly involves a change in diet (with the addition of medication). This is most likely the treatment protocol that your doctor first used with you when you were diagnosed with IBS.

But here's something you may not already know. Did you know that diet and medication are typically only effective for 25% of IBS sufferers? If you are one of the 25% that was able to successfully control your IBS symptoms with changes to your diet and medication then you're actually one of the lucky ones, but then you would probably not be reading this book.

The prognosis for recovery with conventional medical treatment of IBS is poor. In one study of 400 patients[1], only 50% of IBS sufferers reported having **even minor improvements** of their symptoms (such as constipation, diarrhea, and abdominal pain), after one year.

Remember these 400 patients reported only minor improvements after making changes to their diet and taking medication for one year. But what happens after one year? What if we were to look out even further? A study published in 2012 by the American Journal of Gastroenterology[2] followed patients who had been given either hypnotherapy or conventional medical treatment. In this study, clinical remission was defined as having greater than 80% improvement in pain scores. After five years, the study showed that only 20% of the patients receiving conventional medical treatment (diet and medication) were in remission.

Time and time again, research has shown that conventional medical treatment has little proven benefit for IBS sufferers, and yet book after book is written on controlling one's diet. I'm sure that you've gone through this frustration yourself with attempting to make changes to your diet and yet still having problems controlling your IBS symptoms. And if you have been taking medication, either the medication is not working or the side effects are not pleasant.

So wouldn't it be great if there was actually something you could do that had a much higher success rate than just making changes to your diet or taking medication?

If you're like most IBS sufferers, you probably were never told that one of the most researched and best treatments (if not **the** best treatment) for long term control of your IBS symptoms is gut-directed (sometimes called gut-specific) hypnotherapy. There are several research studies that go back over 30 years that validate this. Remember the five year study I discussed a moment ago? How well do you think the patients that received hypnotherapy did? Well after five years, 68% of the patients who received hypnotherapy had more than an 80% improvement in their pain scores. So that's 68% in remission with hypnotherapy compared to 20% in remission with conventional medical treatment. As an IBS sufferer, which treatment program seems better to you?

If you have recently been diagnosed with IBS then you will simply read this book in order, one chapter after the other. Within a short time you will know almost "everything" related to treating IBS, including diet, medication, and other treatment strategies.

If you have been diagnosed with IBS and have been under a doctor's supervision for more than one year, then you will start reading from a different chapter in this book. You will not need all the background information related to what IBS is, is it a problem, what type of IBS you might have, or details about diet and some of the medications that you might be given.

So let's go ahead and look at the next chapter so that you can figure out the best way to use this book based on your individual situation.

4

WHAT'S THE BEST WAY TO USE THIS BOOK?

I'm going to attempt to get into the solution for your IBS symptoms as quickly as possible, based on where you are in your IBS journey. If you're one of the IBS sufferers that already know about diet, medication, and other strategies for treating IBS, and you have been under your doctor's supervision for more than one year, then you can read this book starting from the chapter labeled:

WHAT HAVE WE LEARNED SO FAR?

I'll give you the information as quickly as possible so that you can start making changes to your IBS symptoms. I will only give you the information that I think you'll need so that you can achieve the best results possible. The goal here is to significantly reduce or even eliminate your IBS symptoms.

If you think about it in relationship to your IBS symptoms, current medical treatment has one of two options. The first option is changes to your diet, and the second option is medication. I'm going to suggest that there is a third option. This third option can be used in conjunction with either the first or second option if you wish. As an example if you are currently taking medication, then using this third option will allow the medication to become more effective. If you have made changes to your diet, or if your IBS symptoms seem to be more reactive to certain "trigger" foods, then once again, using the third option can reduce your reactivity to these trigger foods.

The third option can also be used all by itself, and this third option that I'm referring to involves using your mind to make physiological changes in your body. The specific technique that I'll be describing can be traced back (currently more than 30 years) to 1984.

If you think that you have IBS or if you have recently been diagnosed with IBS, then you should start with the chapter that is titled, "What is Irritable Bowel Syndrome?" so that you'll have a very clear picture of what this diagnosis means. You will be told about the typical standard medical treatment for IBS, which includes possible changes to your diet and medications that may be used. I will explain to you what it takes to make a clear diagnosis of IBS, as well as the current treatment strategies. Once your knowledge is up-to-date, then I'll present you with a treatment approach that has been scientifically verified, and yet at the same time is rarely talked about.

If you have been recently diagnosed with IBS, I think it's important for you to understand how difficult it really is to stay up with the current criteria for IBS, and what strategies might work best for you.

Whether you're an IBS sufferer that has been under your doctor's supervision for more than one year, or someone that has been recently diagnosed with IBS, you'll at least want to look at the Table of Contents because there might be information that you'd like to know about, or possibly information that you'd like to review related to your IBS symptoms. Many people are not familiar with all of the different studies that have been done related to current strategies for treating IBS. So it only makes sense that I have included a chapter called, "Current Strategies For IBS."

So again, if you have been diagnosed with IBS and have been under a doctor's supervision for more than one year then look at the Table of Contents, and then you will start reading from the chapter called, "What Have We Learned So Far?"

If you think you have IBS, or have recently been diagnosed with IBS, then take a quick look at the Table of Contents, and continue reading the chapters in order.

5

WHAT IS
IRRITABLE BOWEL SYNDROME?

The first several chapters of this book are basically the, "Everything you wanted to know about IBS but didn't have the time to research" section. After reading these chapters, you will be the equivalent of an "IBS Doctor."

If you're reading this book, you've probably spent a large amount of days and nights with some type of abdominal pain (what some people call cramping), and you also may have bloating, or constipation, or diarrhea, or all of the above. You've probably gone to the doctor many times. You've probably also seen a Gastroenterologist (a gastroenterologist is a medical doctor who specializes in taking care of people with digestive tract problems), and maybe even a psychologist, along with other alternative types of healers. Unfortunately, no matter who you've gone to, you still have had little or no lasting relief.

So if your doctors can find nothing wrong with all this testing, then what do you have? Well, your doctor probably told you that you have something called IBS. "IBS, what's that?"

Let's start by defining Irritable Bowel Syndrome (IBS). IBS is generally classified as a functional disorder characterized by abdominal pain coupled with changes in bowel movements (constipation, diarrhea, or both), where there is no identifiable structural or biochemical cause, such as inflammation, infectious or structural abnormality, but rather an altered physiological function. Think of a functional disorder as one that there is a problem with the functioning of the gut; however, there is no cause that can be seen, measured, or identified.

Apparently IBS was first described in 1812 by an English Physician named William Powell. Powell described what we now call IBS as follows:

> " ... *occasional pain in the intestines and derangement of their powers of digestion, with flatulence and a sense of suffocation*"

Let's look at a few other descriptions from Powell's time up to the early 1900's:

> " ... *spasmodic stricture of the colon – an occasional cause for confinement of the bowels ...*" *Howship 1830*

> " ... *the bowels are at one time constipated, at another lax in the same person ... how the disease has two such different symptoms I do not profess to explain ...*" *Cumming 1849*

> " *Mucous colitis*" *Hurst, 1921*

> "*Neurogenic mucous colitis*" *Bockus et al., 1928*

As you can see there have been many attempts to describe IBS. Still today, the reasons for IBS remain unknown, and because there is no known etiology for IBS, treatments are somewhat arbitrary. This often leads to unsatisfactory treatment outcomes. Originally, conventional medical treatment for IBS included prescribing drugs, and having the patient make dietary changes in hopes of reducing related symptoms.

As we are getting a better understanding of IBS, treatment is moving towards a bio-psycho-social model. In this model, not only are physiological symptoms (such as altered motility, brain-gut dysfunction, and hypersensitivity of the gut) taken into account, but also socio-cultural and psycho-social influences are looked into.

IBS is the most common functional GI disorder, and it is widespread all over the world[1]. It is considered among the top ten reasons that cause people to go to their primary care physician. It is the most common gastrointestinal (GI) disorder seen by GI doctors, encompassing about 30% to 50% of their workload.

IBS cannot be found through something as simple as a blood test, so after a complete history has been taken, patients usually undergo a complete physical examination. This is followed by a series of tests which can include biopsies, CT scan, liver-function tests, x-rays, and colonoscopy, or sigmoidoscopy. Now the good news is that all of those tests probably showed that nothing is wrong.

Some of the "red flags", which **may** rule out IBS that you should inform your physician about, are as follows: anemia, family history of GI cancer, fever, IBD or SPRUCE, new onset of symptoms if you are over 50 years of age, and nocturnal symptoms. In patients with persistent diarrhea, colitis must be ruled out, so a biopsy from the mucosa of the descending colon is often performed. Also your physician should know if you have rectal bleeding, severe constipation, and unexpected weight loss. All this must be done because **a diagnosis of IBS is made by excluding other disorders**.

Some physicians feel uncomfortable making a diagnosis of IBS because they are trained to seek a physical or biological problem. Some physicians even reject the existence of functional GI disorders, which includes IBS. Since these physicians "know that something must be wrong" they pursue unnecessary diagnostic tests.

IBS is not considered a disease; instead, it is a group of symptoms that happen to occur together. The most common symptoms of IBS include abdominal pain or discomfort (which most people would call cramping), bloating, constipation, diarrhea, excess gas, irregular bowel movements, and the frequent and urgent need to use the bathroom.

If a patient shows signs of abdominal pain, and abdominal distension and problems with either frequent constipation or frequent diarrhea (or a combination of the two), and there is no physical problem discovered in the GI tract, then the patient can be diagnosed with IBS.

For some people IBS can be disabling making it impossible to travel to work or attend social events. IBS also causes a great deal of embarrassment along with pain and suffering, but the good news (if there is good news) is that even though a person may have frequent symptoms, IBS does not permanently harm the GI tract and does not lead to other serious diseases.

You may actually have IBS and not know it because previously Irritable Bowel Syndrome went by many names, such as colitis, irritable colon, mucous colitis, nervous colon, nervous stomach, spastic bowel, and spastic colon.

Sometimes IBS is grouped into four subtypes based on a person's usual stool consistency. A patient may be asked to keep a diary to help sub-categorize their symptoms. These subtypes are IBS-C (constipation is predominant), IBS-D (diarrhea is predominant), IBS-A (alternating constipation and diarrhea), and IBS-O (other abdominal symptoms). I will go into these subtypes later in this book.

According to the Rome III Criteria for diagnosis (Rome Foundation, 2006), special attention should be given for the reason behind abdominal pain because it is common to all subtypes of IBS sufferers.

Something that is important to note is that IBS has both physical and mental causes and is not simply in the person's imagination. Since nothing has been found to be wrong, it usually means that the patient's GI tract is highly sensitive. IBS is considered a functional GI disorder. A "functional" diagnosis is intended to reassure the patient that there is no serious disease present, and that the doctor understands the problems that the patient is experiencing. Unfortunately terms like "functional", or terms such as "psychosomatic and somatization", are often misunderstood to mean that the problems are all in the patient's head.

Many doctors also have difficulty explaining functional syndromes to their patients. Functional syndromes are often considered to be related to anxiety, depression, stress, or psychosomatic reactions. The term functional tends to carry a negative connotation, and to the patient, it may imply that their symptoms are imagined, or phony, and not real. These mistaken beliefs also lead to the patient's confusion and frustration.

Because there is no physical proof of the cause of the disorder, many people become frustrated, especially if they are told that, "It's all in your head," or "It's just stress." After enduring a multiplicity of tests, many patients are told that, "There is nothing wrong." Remember that IBS is diagnosed because no visible inflammation or tissue abnormality can be found; this does not mean that there is not a problem; it just means that whatever is wrong is not visible during diagnostic testing.

The truth is that the symptoms that the patient is experiencing are actually real. The patients that have more frequent, or constant and severe GI symptoms, and their symptoms are affecting their lives, it's these patients that are more likely to make an appointment with their doctors.

Imagine for a minute what it must be like to be told that it's just stress, or there's nothing wrong, or that it's just all in your head. For some people that have lived with IBS for an extended period of time without a solution to their problem, it is not unreasonable to suppose that the failure to find a solution to their problem might lead to psychological problems of a purely secondary nature.

If you have IBS then you already know it's a problem, but how bad a problem is it? Is IBS specific to the United States or is it a worldwide problem? Who is likely to get it and how does it compare to other diseases? Let's look at the next chapter to find out.

6

IS IBS REALLY
A PROBLEM?

Let's look at some good news. If you've been given a diagnosis of IBS then you don't have any type of "serious" life threatening disease. How do you know this? You know this because IBS is a diagnosis of exclusion, which means that your doctor has ordered a lot of tests and all the tests came back negative. The bad news is since there is no identifiable cause there is also no identifiable treatment.

You may be wondering if IBS is really a problem at all, so let's look at the worldwide prevalence of IBS. The lowest incidence of IBS is in Iran which reports an incidence of 3.5%. France reports fewer than 10% having IBS. Next, Australia and Germany report that around 12% of the population has IBS, followed by Canada at 13.5%. New Zealand comes in at 17%, with Peru at 18%. China reports 23% and Japan reports 25%, while Nigeria tops the list reporting that 30% of the population has IBS [1, 2].

OK, that's worldwide. Now let's compare IBS to other conditions that you may be more familiar with. In the United States diabetes occurs in about 3% of the population, and asthma occurs in about 4% of the population. Heart disease is prevalent in about 8% of the population and hypertension occurs in about 11% of the population.

As many as one in five people (20%) in the United States (two thirds of which are women) endure Irritable Bowel Syndrome. In women, one in three has symptoms during menstruation, and one in two says that their symptoms worsen during menstruation.

The average onset of IBS for adults is in their twenties, and for children the average onset is typically between 9 to 11 years of age. IBS usually begins before the age of 35 in about 50% of the population, and the symptoms rarely appear after the age of 50. So this is one time that being "old" (like me) is a plus.

IBS is considered the second leading cause of absenteeism in the work place. Can you guess what the first cause is? (Check the last page of this chapter for the answer.) Even though IBS affects so many people, there is relatively little public awareness or appreciation for the problems that it causes. And if that's not bad enough, there is little if any consensus on a clear treatment for IBS. To date, there is no single cure.

IBS is an equal opportunity syndrome, that is, people of all races are affected equally by IBS; however, women are two to three times more likely to be affected than men, but this may be because men are less likely to report the problem. Because men (especially, but some women and children also) are not likely to report GI tract problems, it has been suggested that even greater numbers are not receiving medical care for their symptoms.

The reporting of symptoms usually falls into two categories: those who report that they have had symptoms since childhood, and those who report the onset of symptoms after an accident, illness, or some other particular circumstance. Symptoms can be chronic and appear for months, but they may also just disappear, only to reappear again. For some people, the symptoms can be brutal or even debilitating, and yet for others the symptoms are mild.

Some "lucky" people, (remember about 25%) can control their symptoms with diet, prescribed medications and stress management; however, since IBS can be disabling, others may be unable to work, or even travel short distances, and of course social events are completely out of the question.

Oh, by the way, before we move on, let me answer the question that I asked you before.

THE #1 CAUSE OF ABSENTEEISM
IN THE WORK PLACE IS
THE COMMON COLD.

Are you ready to find out what researchers have found out about what causes IBS, and the risk factors involved? (The cause is not as simple as you might have been led to believe). The next chapter will continue your education so that you can become your own "IBS Doctor."

7

WHAT CAUSES IBS?

We now know that IBS is not considered a disease. It's a worldwide problem that attacks with equal opportunity, but it does strike twice as many women as men. It's considered the second leading cause of absenteeism in the work place. That's all good and fine, but what causes IBS?

Unfortunately researchers have not yet discovered the exact cause of Irritable Bowel Syndrome, but actually that shouldn't come as a big surprise. It turns out that medical research has confirmed that most health care visits are made for common symptoms for which no specific cause can be found. In fact, Dr. Kroenke, M.D. (Indiana University) found the following to be true during his landmark study:

> *"Only 16% of symptoms for which patients consulted with a primary care physician could be medically explained* [1]*."*

IBS has many factors that are linked to it. Many health experts believe that the communication between the brain and the GI tract has broken down, and this imperfect communication leads to the symptoms of IBS. Another theory is that the colon of IBS sufferers is overly sensitive to certain foods and stress. Other researchers have decided that the sensory nerves in the bowel are hypersensitive in people with IBS, and when the bowel wall stretches, they may "overreact."

Scientific studies as well as the clinical experience of gastroenterologists confirm that about one quarter to one third of patients with diarrhea-predominant IBS (IBS-D) reported a previous

---

history of acute gastroenteritis. If you have experienced diarrhea that lasted for more than 21 days compared to people that had diarrhea that lasted less than seven days, then you are 10 times greater at risk for developing IBS.

Research has also shown that patients that have IBS have a greater perception of what's going on in their body. For example, they can feel things in their abdomen, throat, chest, and rectum that other people simply cannot feel. In many cases these feelings are uncomfortable and even painful. Think of it this way, people that have IBS have a lower internal pain threshold than people that do not have IBS. So even normal digestion, and the gas that is produced by the digestion of food, may be experienced as uncomfortable.

Evidence continues to accumulate that implies that IBS is caused by a mixture of biological and psychosocial factors. The "bio-psycho-social" model is described by a number of issues, including abnormal intestinal motility, psychological stress, and visceral hypersensitivity.

These complex mixtures of factors appear to set off the symptoms of IBS. Some of these factors also include hormones, the immune system, and neurotransmitters. Some combinations of these factors appear to interfere with messages between the brain and the GI tract. Any irregular factor causes the bowel to be "irritated" or more sensitive.

The walls of the intestines are lined with layers of muscle that contract and relax at a synchronized pace. This pushes food from your stomach through your GI tract to your rectum. Any miscommunication about the speed or the pressure affects the passage of stool. Sometimes the contractions may be faster and last longer than normal. This causes food to be unnaturally pushed through the intestines too quickly, which causes bloating, gas, and diarrhea. If the passage is too slow then the stools become dry and hard, which leads to constipation.

People who have IBS seem to have an easily upset GI tract, and they react strongly to triggers and variables that do not affect other people. There are two main categories of risk factors that can contribute to IBS. Simply put, those that you can't change, and those that you can change. Some of the triggers that you can't change include:

Age: Only 10% of people over 50 years of age develop IBS. Half of all people with IBS will develop their first symptoms before age 35. (This probably explains why people get so upset when they reach the big three-oh.)

Gender: Compared to men, and probably related to varying hormone levels, women are more than twice as likely to experience IBS symptoms. Their symptoms will typically occur during or around the time of their menstrual periods.

Genetics: It is uncertain whether IBS runs in families; however, studies have shown that IBS is more common in people with family members who have a history of GI problems. Chances are that if IBS runs in your family then you are more likely to experience the symptoms. Remember though that the cause could be environmental or simply because you know what signs to look for.

Health History: Some experts suggest that IBS may be brought on by bacterial infection in the GI tract.

Hormones: Because women are more likely to have (and report) IBS, it stands to reason that hormonal changes may play a role. Post-menopausal women have fewer symptoms compared with women who are still menstruating. Researchers have also found that a woman's IBS symptoms are more pronounced during their menstrual periods, suggesting again that reproductive hormones are playing a role in this condition.

Immune and Nervous Systems: Gut transit speed is regulated by your immune system and your nervous system. These systems control the speed at which food moves through the GI tract. IBS sufferers can suddenly have strong muscle contractions that come and go or even temporarily stop working. Irregular control leads to either constipation or diarrhea. Studies have also shown a relationship between the immune system and GI tract pain sensitivity.

Psychosocial Factors: People who have any type of emotional, physical, or sexual abuse, or psychological conditions (such as anxiety, depression, panic disorder, or post-traumatic stress disorder) have a greater likelihood of having IBS symptoms. The link between these psychosocial factors and the occurrence of IBS is unclear. Researchers believe that people tend to express psychological stress through physical symptoms; in this case the psychological stress would express as IBS symptoms. Researchers typically agree that psychological stress aggravates IBS symptoms. Not only does psychological stress produce GI symptoms in healthy individuals, but the symptoms are worse in patients with IBS.

Sensitivity Level: There is evidence (using balloon inflation) to support that IBS patients have a greater sensitivity to visceral pain. Researchers have found that repetitive balloon inflations in the colon lead to longer and more intense pain intensity in patients with IBS compared to controls. Whatever the reason is, some people have a lower pain threshold to the bowel stretching. Stretching of the bowel can be caused by gas or food moving through the GI tract. The brain just processes these signals from the bowel differently in people with IBS. Even though you can't change your personal sensitivity level, it is possible to learn about and avoid factors that commonly trigger your IBS symptoms (see risk factors that you can change below).

Serotonin Levels: Serotonin (an important neurotransmitter) plays a major role in maintaining a normal digestive system. If serotonin levels are out of balance then bowel problems and IBS symptoms can result. Serotonin is a chemical messenger that transfers messages from one part of your body to another. While only 5% of serotonin is found in the brain, the remaining 95% is located in the GI tract. Abnormal levels of serotonin in the GI tract can result in problems with bowel movement and motility.

Controllable Risk Factors (Things You Can Change)

The other categories of risk factors that can contribute to IBS are things that you can change. These controllable risk factors will probably lower the intensity or frequency of your IBS symptoms and include:

Eating Habits: Eating a large meal causes abdominal distention, which can contribute to IBS symptoms. If you need to consume more calories, eat smaller more frequent meals, which can help reduce discomfort.

Emotional Choices: Bottling up your emotions also creates digestive problems for a person that is prone to IBS. Emotions such as unresolved anger, anxiety, blaming yourself or others, excessive fear or worry, feelings of helplessness, frustration, grief, guilt, lack of a loving relationship, and self-criticism, will all have negative effects on your digestive system.

Research has shown that expressing painful feelings that result in tears from anger, fear, and sadness, differ in composition from tears produced by chemical irritants. It turns out that emotional tears remove toxins from the body.

Other studies have shown that patients in the early stages of malignant melanoma were able to stimulate their immune system increasing their natural killer cell activity by expressing anger at having the disease. It is repressed anger, not expressed anger in appropriate ways, which damages your body and psyche.

Your inability to remove unresolved negative emotions (such as anger, or sadness, or fear, or guilt) in many cases was acquired in childhood. You learned that expressing negative emotions was unacceptable. As a child you simply didn't have the words to express yourself, let alone the freedom to do so, so the negative emotions stayed locked inside your body. Expressing your negative feelings in the right environment is extremely healing.

Food: Most patients are certain that some type of food allergy is responsible for their IBS symptoms, and many complain that eating makes their symptoms worse. Many patients have tried high-fiber diets despite compelling evidence that high-fiber diets result in patients being made worse rather than better. Even though exclusion diets produce very disappointing results and no specific food has been linked with IBS, certain foods and beverages can cause symptoms to flare up. Alcohol, barley, carbonated beverages, chocolate, coffee, dairy products, food or drinks that contain caffeine, fatty foods, rye, soda, spicy foods, wheat, some fruits, sugar-free gum, and some vegetables, **may** make symptoms worse. As a rule, people with food sensitivity do not have clinical signs of food allergies, especially related to IBS. Some researchers have suggested that IBS symptoms may occur because of poor absorption of sugars or bile acids.

Lifestyle Choices: Things like lack of exercise, lack of play or recreation, and smoking, as well as inadequate preventative care, can greatly affect your IBS symptoms.

Medications: Patients are typically given antispasmodics, laxatives, or anti-diarrheals as appropriate, and even more recently, receptor-modifying drugs are also given. Several types of medications can bring on IBS symptoms. Talk to your doctor or pharmacist about finding a different medication if you think the medication you're taking is responsible for your symptoms.

Weight: Research has demonstrated that gastrointestinal pain is related to higher Body Mass Index (BMI). BMI measures the relative percentages of fat and muscle mass in the human body, and the result is used as an index of obesity. Researchers measured transit time verses BMI and found that being overweight was associated with increased risk of having IBS symptoms. Eating a healthy diet and exercising regularly can help you lose weight and therefore reduce IBS symptoms.

Stress Levels. Stress, especially uncontrolled chronic stress, can promote colon spasms in people with IBS. The colon is partly controlled by the autonomic nervous system, and it also has many nerves that connect it to the brain. These nerves not only control normal contractions in the colon, but during times of minor disputes or stress, these nerves can cause abdominal discomfort. People that have IBS usually have an excessively responsive colon, and any stress makes the person perceive sensations in the colon as unpleasant.

We all know that it is nearly impossible to control all the stressors in our life; however, we do have direct control over how we choose to respond to situations that cause stress. Most people with IBS notice that their symptoms are aggravated during stressful events. And for some people something as simple as a change in their daily routine causes them to stress out.

We know that the immune system is affected by stress, and there is some evidence that suggests that IBS is affected by the immune system. Although stress may aggravate IBS symptoms, it is not the root cause of the symptoms.

For most if not all IBS sufferers, stress management should become an important part of their life. Different stress management options include:

Adequate sleep

Counseling and support

Deep breathing

Reducing stressful situations in your life

Regular exercise (even walking works)

Relaxation training

Self-Hypnosis

Yoga

So that you can finally understand how difficult it is to diagnose IBS, in the next chapter you'll be presented with a number of case histories. I want you to see how good you would be at coming up with an accurate diagnosis of IBS, especially since the criteria continue to change and evolve. OK, so put on your doctor's smock and let's see how well you can do with your new patients, Tracy, Bob, Christine, John, and Laurie.

8

HOW IS
IBS DIAGNOSED?

So far your education consists of knowing that there is no physical problem discovered in the GI tract. You also now know about controllable risk factors as well as uncontrollable risk factors. It's now time to learn how IBS is diagnosed.

So that you can better understand the difficulty in diagnosing IBS, I'm going to present you with the title of "IBS Doctor," (congratulations!!!) but only while you're reading this book.

Let's assume that you're starting a new job as an "IBS Doctor" at a medical clinic. This is your first day and you have the written case histories of the patients that you will be seeing (these case histories might even be very similar to your own situation). The following patients want your "expert" opinion and diagnosis with the problem that they are having. It will be up to you to determine if they have IBS or not. So if you're ready, let all your newly acquired "IBS Doctor" knowledge settle in and let's look at a few "simple" case histories of people with bowel problems.

"Tracy" is a 42-year-old trial attorney. She had been in a fender-bender about six months ago, and had suffered some minor injuries, but the injuries were bad enough for her to be hospitalized. Tracy had a slight concussion and some minor cuts and abrasions, so she was kept overnight for observation. About one week after being released from the hospital, Tracy began having stomach cramps and as she described it, "I have very loose bowels and I'm in the bathroom way too many times each day. Right before my bowel movements, my stomach cramps get worse, but I do feel much better afterwards."

Tracy wondered if she had picked-up some kind of bug while in the hospital. She continued having symptoms for about one month before she finally went to her doctor. She asked her doctor about possibly picking up a bug in the hospital, and her doctor told her that it was unlikely. To help with her loose bowels, her doctor suggested that she add more fiber to her diet.

So "IBS Doctor" does Tracy have IBS or not?

Let me add to your knowledge as an "IBS Doctor." It turns out that there is no specific test for IBS; diagnostic tests are used to rule out other diseases. In order to rule out other diseases, a complete medical history is done that starts with a thorough physical examination including a description of the patient's symptoms. Other tests may include blood tests (to rule out infection), stool samples (to rule out parasite infection or bleeding in the gut), and x-rays. The doctor may look inside the patient's colon by inserting a small, flexible tube with a camera on the end of it through the anus. This procedure is called a sigmoidoscopy, or colonoscopy and this procedure is looking for lesions or other abnormalities in the intestines.

Even though there is no specific test for IBS, symptom-based criteria helps steer the diagnostic and treatment method. More and more, symptom-based criteria are accepted within gastroenterology, and are already used in psychiatry (DSM V) and rheumatology.

Many different diseases and disorders mimic IBS symptoms, including bowel diseases such as Crohn's disease, ulcerative colitis, and endometriosis. Food allergies, inflammatory colon cancer, and gluten intolerance disorders such as celiac disease also have similar symptoms. These other diseases must all be conclusively ruled out before a diagnostic of IBS can be made.

OK, since we have now increased your knowledge of how to diagnose IBS, based on this latest information, see if using this new information is enough to diagnose Tracy with IBS. Since you're new at being an "IBS Doctor," (and to make the diagnosis a little easier for you, after all it is your first day) you have just come across another page in Tracy's case history. So let's start reading again from the beginning.

Tracy is a 42-year-old trial attorney. She had been in a fender-bender about six months ago, and had suffered some minor injuries, but the injuries were bad enough for her to be hospitalized. Tracy had a slight concussion and some minor cuts and abrasions, so she was kept overnight for observation.

About one week after being released from the hospital, Tracy began having stomach cramps and as she described it, "I have very loose bowels and I'm in the bathroom way too many times each day. Sometimes I look like I'm three months pregnant. Right before my bowel movements, my stomach cramps get worse, but I do feel much better afterwards."

Tracy wondered if she had picked-up some kind of bug while in the hospital. She continued having symptoms for about one month before she finally went to her doctor. She asked her doctor about possibly picking up a bug in the hospital, and her doctor told her that it was unlikely. To help with her loose bowels, her doctor suggested that she add more fiber to her diet.

Tracy went back to her doctor after two weeks and reported that even with the extra fiber her diarrhea was as bad as ever. Tracy's doctor ran test after test after test, but the entire battery of tests came back normal. No blood in the stools, no inflammation, no food allergies, no lesions, no nothing. Everything looked fine.

So you're the "IBS Doctor," do you now have enough information to diagnosis Tracy with IBS or not, and how do you know one way or the other? I mean, what are the criteria? Oh yeah, that's right, you do need some criteria to do a proper diagnosis.

In 1978, Manning, et al.,[1] first developed the diagnostic criteria for IBS. This was the criteria that was used to diagnosis IBS until around 1988 when Rome I came out. The Rome Foundation (**www.romecriteria.org**) brings together worldwide information from clinicians and scientists to classify functional gastrointestinal disorders (FGIDs).

Both Manning and Rome consist of a collection of symptoms that, in the absence of biochemical or structural disorders of the GI tract, allow for the diagnosis of IBS.

If all tests results are negative, then the doctor may diagnose IBS based on the symptoms alone. The first established diagnostic guideline was the Manning Criteria, and then came the Rome I, Rome II, and we now have the Rome III Criteria (and the committee is working on Rome IV).

Depending on which guideline is being used, you may or may not be diagnosed with IBS. In a study of over 40,000 people done in 2003 by Hungin et al.,[2] 6.5% met the Manning criteria, 4.2% met the Rome I criteria, and only 2.9% met the Rome II criteria. This is because the Manning criteria are based on pain relieved by bowel movement, onset of pain linked to more frequent bowel movements, and looser stools with the onset of pain, where Rome I and the later Rome II criteria are more refined, and include the duration of symptoms within their definitions, Rome II being the more (if not too) restrictive.

Between August 1975 and May 1976, Manning and his colleagues devised criteria which distinguished IBS from organic diseases of the GI tract. They used a questionnaire containing 15 symptoms (see below) thought to be typical of IBS. Seventeen to twenty-six months later, data was reviewed on 106 patients that were originally referred to gastroenterology or surgery clinics with abdominal pain or a change in bowel habit or both. A definite diagnosis was reached in 79 of the 106 patients, of which IBS was diagnosed in 32 patients, and 33 patients had organic disease.

The original Manning Criteria basically was interested in symptoms like abdominal bloating, pain related to bowel movements, altered bowel habits, emptying, and mucus in the patient's stool. You as an "IBS Doctor" should pay attention to the symptoms that your patient is describing. The 15 symptoms in the questionnaire looked similar to the following:

1. At the onset of pain - looser stools
2. At the onset of pain - more frequent bowel movements
3. At the onset of pain - harder stools
4. At the onset of pain - less frequent bowel movements
5. Often after a bowel movement pain is reduced
6. Visible distension
7. Feeling of distension
8. Mucus in the stools
9. Often having a feeling of incomplete emptying
10. Bowel movement before breakfast
11. Nocturnal bowel movement
12. Urgency of defecation
13. Pain worse after bowel movement
14. Pain eased with flatus
15. Greater than two bowel movements between meals

It was later discovered that this questionnaire was not specific enough and was unreliable for use with men who have IBS. Results from the study concluded that six cardinal symptoms discriminated the painful variant of IBS from organic bowel disease. IBS is defined as the symptoms given below with no duration of symptoms described. The key symptoms turned into the Manning Criteria and are as follows:

1. Onset of pain linked to more frequent bowel movements
2. Looser stools associated with onset of pain
3. Pain relieved by passage of stool
4. Noticeable abdominal bloating
5. Sensation of incomplete evacuation more than 25% of the time
6. Diarrhea with mucus more than 25% of the time

Mucus in the stools can be a sign of Crohns disease, inflammation, or Irritable Bowel Syndrome. Only the diagnosis of a medical doctor can determine the cause of mucus in the stools.

According to Manning's information, four symptoms were significantly more common among patients with IBS. These four symptoms are as follows:

1. Onset of pain linked to more frequent bowel movements
2. Pain relieved by passage of stool
3. Noticeable abdominal bloating
4. Diarrhea with mucus more than 25% of the time

The more symptoms that were present, the more likely it was that patients had Irritable Bowel Syndrome, but a threshold of three symptoms is the most commonly used.

So as a new "IBS Doctor," if you were using only the Manning criteria, can Tracy be diagnosed with IBS?

Let's look at another case history. Get ready to meet Bob.

"Bob" worked for a large company as a local salesman for computers. Bob had been a jock most of his life, and at the age of 36 he was in great physical shape. Bob and a bunch of his friends at work were on the company's softball team and he was one of their best players.

During one of the play-off games, Bob twisted his knee and had to be removed from the game (by the way they won). His knee still hurt after a few days and wasn't getting any better, so he finally decided to have it looked at. The doctor decided that Bob had torn his meniscus and that he would need surgery.

Bob said that the surgery was no big deal. They had him under general anesthesia for just long enough to insert a small camera, a tube for water (which puffed his knee up), and a small "roto-router" device for shaving the meniscus. Bob said that everything went as planned and he would have plenty of time to recover before softball season was back. The doctor prescribed antibiotics and pain medication for Bob.

Bob was doing fine, until after about ten days when his stomach started growling; he felt bloated, and his bowel movements become a little loose. Pretty soon he had diarrhea, and sometimes he barely (and I mean barely) made it to the bathroom. He knew when his stomach started to cramp that it was smart to head toward the bathroom. Bob had mixed feelings about being in the bathroom so much because it was like being on a see-saw with the pain, that is, cramps before and feel better after.

After a week of this Bob had enough and called his doctor. The doctor told him that it could be a delayed reaction to the antibiotics and pain medication. His doctor told him to give it another week for the medications to be completely out of his system and to give him a call in a week or so to let him know what was happening. He also told Bob to add some fiber to his diet to reduce the diarrhea.

Bob did a fair amount of traveling, although not very far, after all he was a local salesman for computers. But now before he made a business trip to see a potential client he mapped-out where bathrooms were located along the way. If he was required to attend a meeting at work he would sit near the door, just in case he had to leave quickly.

The extra week came and went but Bob still had diarrhea. He went back to the doctor, but even with all the tests that were run, they couldn't find anything wrong. Bob's doctor knew that Bob was in a high stress job because after all Bob was one of his company's top salesmen. So the doctor told Bob to relax more and take care of himself. That was nine months ago, and Bob said not much has changed. He still has almost no control over his bowels, but he has become an expert at coming up with excuses for why he can't go to parties or attend other events. Unfortunately, Bob had to give up one of his joys and had to quit the company's softball team.

Before you make a determination about Bob, and does he have IBS according to the Manning criteria, let's take a moment to follow the "new" criteria, called Rome I that was being developed around 1984 or so.

Another Set of Guidelines

Around 1984, discussions for further guidelines for the diagnosis of IBS where held by the 12th International Congress of Gastroenterology. A team was set up in 1986 to develop the Rome I guidelines, and a draft of these guidelines was sent to sixteen people from seven different countries that were noted for their research in IBS. Once their comments were received back, the new draft was presented at the 13th International Congress in Rome in 1988.

This is what the draft looked like:

Continuous or recurrent symptoms of abdominal pain (or discomfort) that is:

Relieved by defecation AND/OR

Associated with a change in stool or consistency

Plus disturbed defecation (must have two or more of the following):

Altered stool frequency (more than three per day or less than three per week)

Altered stool form (lumpy, hard or watery, loose)

Altered Stool Passage (feeling of incomplete evacuation, straining or urgency)

Passage of mucus

Bloating or feeling of abdominal distention

A committee was set up to break down IBS symptoms into subgroups. The project was expanded, and the committee ended up classifying the functional GI disorders into 21 entities. Pain became a requirement and additional committees were set up. In 1992, the Rome I Criteria was published.

OK, you're the "IBS Doctor," did Bob have IBS according to the Manning criteria? And what about the Rome I criteria? See if according to the Rome I draft above, you can determine if Bob has IBS or not. Is it possible to have IBS according to the Manning criteria, but not the Rome I criteria? Or is it possible to have IBS according to the Rome I criteria, but not the Manning criteria? You're the "IBS Doctor," what do you do if he has IBS according to one set of criteria but not the other?

The Rome committee continued revising the criteria for IBS. We don't have time right now to continue your education, because your next patient just entered the waiting room. Go ahead and take a look at Christine's case history so you can continue improving your skills.

"Christine" was 38 years old but says she felt more like 83. In her late 20's, she started having severe abdominal pain, but since her symptoms would come and go, it was hard for her to figure out what was causing the pain. Sometimes she would have abdominal pain right around her period, and other times, just out of the blue, she would be incapacitated with cramps that would last about seven days.

At the same time the pain occurred she would experience constipation. It was as if she just didn't need to have a bowel movement. During these times, if she had more than one bowel movement per week that was a lot.

She just figured that this was "normal" for her, but a close friend told her otherwise, so she finally went to her doctor about it. Her doctor ran test after test but couldn't find a reason for the pain. So (as usual) her doctor suggested that she watch her diet, and also prescribed pain medications and a laxative.

Christine was given a lot of medications but nothing seemed to work. The medications gave Christine some short-term relief, but the pain by no means left completely. Christine had always liked spicy foods, and when she went to a nutritionist to help her with her diet it was the first thing to go. But no matter what she ate or didn't eat her symptoms always came back.

OK "Doc," what is your diagnosis of Christine's problem? Does it fit the Manning criteria or the Rome I criteria? Since you're now Christine's medical doctor, would you diagnosis her with IBS?

Let's go back to the Rome committee. Work on the Rome committee continued to expand the information on IBS and GI disorders, and members from basic science, pediatric physiology, and psychosocial were included. The committees produced a series of articles which were included as a supplement in *Gut* 4: 16-26,

1999. In 2000, Rome II Criteria was published from this expanded data.

Below are the diagnostic conditions for IBS according to the Rome II Criteria. After reading the criteria, go back to Bob's case history and determine if Bob had IBS according to the Rome II criteria.

Patient should have at least 3 months continuous or recurrent symptoms in the previous 12 months of:

1) Abdominal discomfort or pain and must have two out of three of the following:

   a. Relieved with defecation.

   b. Onset associated with a change in consistency of stool.

   c. Onset associated with a change in frequency of stool.

AND

2. Two or more of the following, at least a quarter of occasions or days:

   a. Altered stool frequency:

      i) More than 3 bowel movements per day, **OR**

      ii) Less than 3 bowel movements per week

   b. Altered stool form:

      i) Lumpy / hard, **OR**

      ii) Loose / watery stool

   c. Altered stool passage:

      i) Feeling of incomplete evacuation, **OR**

      ii) Straining, **OR**

      iii) Urgency, **OR**

d. Passage of mucus.

e. Bloating or feeling of abdominal distension.

Remember as an "IBS Doctor" you need to keep up with new criteria, so keep in mind the Rome II criteria, because another patient has entered the waiting room. Let's become familiar with John as we investigate another case history.

"John" was a 25-year-old history student who decided to take some time away from his studies to travel. During his travels in Asia he had a mild case of food poisoning and was vomiting, and he also had a mild case of the runs. In Africa he contracted a staph infection. John was treated with the oral form of Vancomycin, and all seemed better; however, within a short time, John developed diarrhea and had to cut his travels short. When John got back to the states, his doctor told him that diarrhea was a common side effect of Vancomycin. He told his doctor that since having the staph infection and traveling for the last four months, he was having loose stools more often now, probably once a week, but the rest of the week his bowel movements were normal. He said it was sort of weird that after each bowel movement his discomfort simply went away. John also said that it seemed to flair-up when he had any kind of carbonated drinks.

What's your diagnosis of John according to the Rome II criteria? After you figure out John's diagnosis, let's look at your next patient's case history.

"Laurie" is 28 and she had her second baby last year. Laurie described her first pregnancy as "easy," but her second baby was a completely different story. As Laurie described it, "Lots of pain, lots of pushing, followed by lots more pain, and a lot more pushing." About one month after the baby was born Laurie started complaining that she didn't feel like her old self. Her main complaint was bloating and abdominal pain with really loose stools. After hearing this, according to the paper work you have from Laurie's previous doctor, her doctor immediately diagnosed Laurie with IBS.

Was Laurie's previous doctor correct in his diagnosis? According to the Rome II criteria, does Laurie have IBS? You're Laurie's new "IBS Doctor," what would your diagnosis be?

If these patients were too easy for you, then let's change the guidelines one more time because two more of your new patients just walked in the door. In a moment you'll be introduced to Sally and Alisha, and you'll find that they both had an interesting type of treatment that worked well for them. See what you think about their case histories.

9

MAKING SIMPLER
IBS GUIDELINES

The expansion from Rome II to a simpler Rome III Criteria started in 2001. Most of the Rome II committees stayed together, and culture, functional abdominal pain, gender, pharmacology, society and the patient, and two pediatric committees were added. In 2006, the Rome III publication was released by the American College of Gastroenterology Functional Disorders Task Force (American Gastroenterological Association, 2006). The "main" difference between Rome II and Rome III is that the time frame was changed. Moreover, the single classification was based on stool consistency.

Changes from Rome II to Rome III not only reflected committee recommendations derived from new data, but changes in the categories and criteria were also made as follows:

The time frame change was changed. Originally in the Rome II criteria, a patient had to have 12 weeks of symptoms over a 12 month period. Rome III reduced that restriction and recommended that symptoms start six months before diagnosis and be currently active for three months.

Rome III revised IBS sub-typing. The committees suggested that constipation, diarrhea, and mixed subtypes, should be classified based on stool consistency. IBS-C and IBS-D bowel sub-typing used in Rome II are still acceptable to use for subtyping.

Rome III classified Functional Gastro-Intestinal Disorders (FGIDs) into six symptom-based major diagnostic criteria categories for adults (with 28 categories in all). FGID symptoms correlate to mixtures of quite a few known physiological determinants: IBS is multifaceted and results from a combination of alterations of bacterial flora, CNS-ENS dysregulation, dysmotility, mucosal immune dysregulation, and visceral hypersensitivity.

Here are the six major diagnostic criteria categories for adults:

A: Esophageal

B: Gastroduodenal

C: Bowel

D: Functional abdominal pain syndrome (FAPS)

E: Biliary

F: Anorectal

There is also a pediatric system that is classified by age range first, and then by symptom pattern or area of symptom location.

Each category has specific clinical features and contains several disorders. Category C, which is functional bowel disorders, is anatomically attributed to the small bowel, colon, and rectum. Category C includes IBS (C1), functional bloating (C2), functional constipation (C3), and functional diarrhea (C4). It is worthwhile to note that some symptoms, such as bloating, constipation, diarrhea, and pain, overlap across disorders.

> *IBS is specifically distinct in its definition,*
> *which is pain associated with*
> *change in bowel habit.*

This is different from functional diarrhea (C4), which is distinguished by loose stools and no pain, or functional bloating (C2), in which there is no change in bowel habit.

So the Rome III definition for Irritable Bowel Syndrome (IBS) is pain associated with change in bowel habit. It's symptoms of recurrent abdominal pain, or uncomfortable sensations not described as pain, must have occurred for the previous three months with symptoms starting at least six months prior to diagnosis. These changes in bowel habit must occur at least three days per month for the last three months and two or more of the following must be present:

1. Pain is relieved (that is, there is less pain) by having a bowel movement

2. Onset of pain is related to a change in frequency of stool

3. Onset of pain is related to a change in the appearance of stool

Although the Rome III Criteria has established both IBS-M (mixed symptoms) and IBS-U (Unsubtyped symptoms), some physicians find it useful to use the following earlier IBS sub-divisions:

IBS-C = Constipation-predominant

IBS-D = Diarrhea-predominant

IBS-A = Alternating constipation and diarrhea

IBS-A = Is the same as IBS-M

IBS-O = Other abdominal symptoms

IBS-O = Is the same as IBS-U

Studies show that only a few GPs follow these criteria, but with these criteria now clearly defined, a medical doctor should be able to diagnose IBS safely with fewer tests. Bleeding, fever, persistent severe pain, and weight loss, are NOT symptoms of IBS and may indicate other problems.

OK, as an "IBS Doctor" you're now able to understand the Rome III criteria for IBS. So let's look at a couple more cases that have come your way.

"Sally" is a 35-year-old high school math teacher. Sally went to her primary care physician complaining of being tired all the time and having cramps (abdominal pain) most days of the month. But her main complaint was that she just didn't seem to have any control over her bowel movements. Sometimes they were "normal," then sometimes they would be runny for a few days, and other times there would be no bowel movements at all for a week. Sally said that this was pretty new, but it had been happening on and off for the last year, but over the last four months the problem has been pretty consistent. She also said that when she has diarrhea the pain occurs more often, but she always feels better after having a bowel movement.

Her doctor told Sally to keep a food diary and suggested that she take laxatives if she was constipated and to add fiber to her diet to stop the diarrhea. Sally continued going to her primary care physician many times with no success, so her primary care physician sent her to a gastroenterologist.

Sally's gastroenterologist ran lots and lots of tests but could find nothing wrong. Sally was put on high dosages of multiple medications that she reported as having way too many side effects. Nothing was working for her, and although Sally's primary care physician did not think that Sally had IBS, her gastroenterologist diagnosed Sally with IBS, and ahead of his time he sent Sally to see a hypnotherapist that was familiar with treating IBS.

When Sally came for her first hypnotherapy session she said the laxatives had helped her constipation, but even with the rest of the medications she still had runny, watery stools, sometimes many times a day.

Sally was asked to rate her symptoms on a scale of zero to ten, with ten being as bad as it can get and zero being normal. She rated her symptoms as follows: abdominal pain 8, bloating 6, diarrhea 8, and fatigue 8.

At the beginning of the fourth session (having had three hypnotherapy sessions) Sally rated the same symptoms as follows:

abdominal pain 4 or so; bloating maybe 3, diarrhea 3 or 4, and fatigue as almost normal (0 or 1).

By the end of the seventh hypnotherapy session, Sally reported that all her symptoms were either a one or a zero. She reported these symptom improvements even though she was a little stressed-out because her father had recently gone into the hospital after having a small stroke.

So did Sally have IBS according to the Rome III criteria or not? And why did the hypnotherapy have such an effect on her symptoms?

Let's look at our last case history as you keep the Rome III criteria in mind.

"Alisha" was 18 and was just entering junior college. She was a lot of fun to be around and attended numerous social events. None of her friends realized the embarrassment she suffered almost every day.

Alisha had digestive problems since she was a small child. Alisha's mom said she was a sensitive child because she had a "nervous stomach." Alisha missed many days of school because she was inclined to have either constipation or diarrhea.

During the times when she was in her "constipation mode," Alisha said that she would go for days without having even one bowel movement. There was never a time that she remembered that she had a bowel movement each day or even every other day. She knew that "constipation mode" was coming because she would have cramps before trying to have a bowel movement. She could sit on the toilet for 30 minutes at a time and nothing would happen, except maybe passing a large amount of gas. One of her fears was that she would pass gas during class and everyone would know that it was her.

During the times when she was in her "diarrhea mode," Alisha said that she literally had to run to the bathroom as many as five times each day. "Diarrhea mode" usually lasts for three to four days at a time. Sometimes at school she would have an episode of uncontrolled diarrhea in the girl's bathroom. She said the smell was embarrassing, and the sounds were even worse, but at least she felt better afterwards.

Alisha had seen many doctors starting in her early teens, including a gastroenterologist. Her doctors had run tests, and her gastroenterologist ran even more tests, but none of her doctors could find anything wrong. They figured that she must be allergic to some type of food, or that it was just stress. The GI doctor did tell her that she probably had a condition called Irritable Bowel Syndrome.

Her doctor gave her a list of foods that may cause problems, which turned out to be most of what she was eating. The doctor told her to watch out for foods or drinks containing caffeine, sugar, and carbonated beverages (there went soft drinks). He also said to avoid red meat and cheese (there goes pizza and cheeseburgers). After he told here to restrict her chocolate intake she quit listening.

Alisha was put on high dosages of multiple medications, all of which had really bad side effects. But maybe even worse than the side effects, the medications didn't seem to do much of anything for her symptoms. Alisha went into a deep level of depression and dropped out of school.

When Alisha came for her first hypnotherapy session, she was still taking multi-medications, and was now on a medication for her depression. She was a little apprehensive about hypnosis, but was willing to try anything.

Alisha rated her symptoms as follows: abdominal pain 9, bloating 6, diarrhea 9, fatigue 9, and sadness (depression) was an 8.

At the beginning of the fifth session (having had four hypnotherapy sessions), Alisha rated the same symptoms as follows: abdominal pain 6 or so; bloating maybe 4, diarrhea 5 or 6, fatigue 6, and sadness was the most improved and she rated it as a 3 or 4.

By the end of the seventh hypnotherapy session, Alisha reported her symptoms as follows: abdominal pain 3 or 4; bloating 2, diarrhea 2 or 3, fatigue 3, and sadness down to a 1 or 2, so she had asked her doctor if she could reduce her depression medication.

Alisha continued for three more sessions (ten hypnotherapy sessions in total). At the end of all the sessions, Alisha reported that her symptoms were either a one or a zero, and when she felt stressed out they would rise to a 1 or 2. It was decided to do hypnotherapy "tune-ups" once a month until she felt that she was back to her old self.

OK that was pretty good for your first day as an "IBS Doctor". Let's read on and find out if you agree with the conclusions that other "Doctors" came up with.

10

POSSIBLE CONCLUSIONS FROM THE CASE HISTORIES

Since you are now a highly educated "IBS Doctor," see if you agree with the following possible conclusions.

Our first case history was about our 42-year-old trial attorney named Tracy. We know that after Tracy's "minor" traffic accident, she ended up having stomach cramps (pain) and loose bowels (diarrhea) which caused her numerous trips to the bathroom each day. She described her pain as getting worse before her bowel movements, and relieved after.

Her doctor added fiber to her diet but ran no tests, so a diagnosis of IBS is premature.

We added a little more information to the second Tracy case history. In this case history, Tracy went back to her doctor two weeks later at which time he ran a battery of tests. All tests came back normal. We know that IBS is a diagnostic of exclusion, and the doctor conclusively ruled out other diseases. Technically, I hadn't given you any criteria for what IBS is, so you really can't diagnose IBS yet. You do know what Tracy does not have, but with no other criteria you can't really say what she does have.

Later, I gave you the first diagnostic criteria for IBS developed by Manning, et al. So if we were using the Manning criteria, can Tracy be diagnosed with IBS?

Remember the doctor excluded "all" other diseases. Tracy does mention abdominal bloating (I look like I'm three months pregnant). There is no direct discussion about incomplete emptying because she has diarrhea. She does have pain right before her bowel movements, and since she has loose stools, then pain would be associated with looser stools. Also pain eases after her bowel movement. If a doctor was familiar with IBS, he would probably diagnose Tracy with IBS.

The next case history was about Bob, our 36-year-old softball playing computer salesman. Bob ended up having bowel problems after his knee surgery. Even with all the tests that were run, no reason could be found for Bob's symptoms. There was abdominal bloating, and like Tracy there is no direct mention of incomplete emptying because he has diarrhea. Bob does have pain before and feels better after his bowel movements, and the doctor made no comment about any mucus in the stools, which could have ruled out IBS if it was Crohns disease, or inflammation. So according to the Manning criteria, Bob can be diagnosed with IBS.

Next, I gave you the diagnostic criteria according to Rome I. Let's take a moment and evaluate Bob's case history and determine if Bob meets the criteria for IBS according to Rome I. I think what you're going to find is that the doctor needs to ask specific questions to make a determination of IBS.

Bob definitely has recurrent abdominal pain relieved with defecation. According to Rome I that is enough to diagnosis IBS (with the assumption that all tests are normal). So in Bob's case he can be diagnosed with IBS by both the Manning criteria and the Rome I criteria.

Next, I gave you the diagnostic criteria according to Rome II. According to the Rome II criteria, did Bob have IBS?

This one is simple (I hope). Rome II added time in the criteria for diagnosing IBS, specifically,

> "Patient should have at least 3 months continuous or recurrent symptoms in the previous 12 months."

Bob's problem was pretty recent. He first starting having bowel problems about ten days after his surgery, waited a week to call his doctor, and his doctor told him to wait an extra week to let the medications "clear" out of his system. Bob went back to the doctor to have tests run, but no problem was found. So at the most Bob had the symptoms for about one month. At this point Bob never returned to the doctor and is living with the problem. So Bob does not meet the Rome II criteria of "at least 3 months of recurrent symptoms;" however, if Bob had gone back to his doctor any time after 3 months of having the symptoms (he is still living with no control over his bowels nine months later), then his doctor would be able to diagnosis Bob with IBS according to the Rome II criteria.

Our next case history was about 33-year-old, Christine. Let's first determine if she has IBS according to the Manning Criteria.

First, her doctor ruled out the possibility of other diseases (her doctor ran test after test but couldn't find a reason for the pain). Christine experienced pain at the same time when she would have constipation, but there was no noticeable bloating, or pain relieved by passage of stool. She also didn't have loose stools or diarrhea. It sure looks like according to the Manning Criteria, Christine does not have IBS, so now let's look at the Rome I.

Christine did not complain of bloating or feeling any abdominal distension, and there is no discussion of the passage of mucus. She does have recurrent abdominal pain (her symptoms would come and go) associated with a change in frequency or consistency of stool (at the same time the pain occurred, she would experience constipation). She does have disturbed defecation where the frequency of bowel movements changed (during these times, if she had more than one bowel movement per week that was a lot). She did have hard stools (constipated). So it looks like according to Rome I criteria, Christine does have IBS.

Did our 25-year-old history student, John, have IBS according to the Rome II criteria? Let's take a look. The first thing we notice is that John does meet the time criteria. He told his doctor that he was having loose stools for the last four months. His abdominal discomfort is relieved with defecation. John only has loose stools about once a week, so he doesn't meet the criteria for more than 3 bowel movements per day. Again since he only has loose stools about once a week, and the rest of the time his bowels are normal, then he does not meet the criteria for loose stools a quarter of occasions or days. Also there was no discussion about straining, or urgency, or bloating, or abdominal distention. So I think based on this information, and according to the Rome II criteria, John does not have IBS.

Now how about our new mom Laurie? Laurie's doctor immediately diagnosed her with IBS. This one is really easy. Think about it. First off no tests were run, and since IBS is a diagnosis of exclusion, "all" other diseases and causes must be ruled out. Also, the only time frame we have is that one month after the baby was born Laurie started complaining about bloating, abdominal pain, and loose stools. So Laurie does not meet the three month requirement. According to this information, it is extremely premature to make a diagnosis of IBS.

Next you were given information to help you understand the Rome III criteria for IBS. So let's look at our 35-year-old high school math teacher, Sally. She complained of abdominal pain most days of the month, and her bowel movements varied from normal, to runny, to none. Sally also said that this had been happening on and off for the last year, and over the last four months the problem has been pretty consistent. So we know that Sally meets the criteria for recurrent abdominal pain at least the previous three months, with symptoms starting at least six months ago. She has changes in bowel habit at least three days per month (sometimes they were "normal", then sometimes they would be runny for a few days, and other times there would be no bowel movements at all for a week). And these changes have occurred for at least the last three months (happening on and off for the last year). Sally also has pain relieved by a bowel movement, and her onset of pain is related to a change in the frequency of stool (remember she said that when she has diarrhea the pain occurs more often, but she always feels better after having a bowel movement.) Sally's gastroenterologist ruled out other diseases (lots and lots of tests and could find nothing wrong). So from the information we have, Sally should have been diagnosed with IBS.

Our last case history is about our 18-year-old college student named Alisha. Alisha has had bowel problems starting in her early teens, which fulfills the six months prior to diagnosis criteria, and continues to have problems (she's 18 now) which fulfills the previous three months requirement. Her doctors and her gastroenterologist ran tests, but none of them could find any disease. In "constipation mode" she goes for days without having a bowel movement, and "diarrhea mode" usually lasts for three to four days at a time, so she meets the changes in bowel habit at least three days per month for the last three months requirement. Before "constipation mode" hit, she would experience cramps, and in "diarrhea mode" she would feel better after her bowel movements. So using all the information that Alisha gave her doctors, her GI doctor was right when he said that she probably had a condition called Irritable Bowel Syndrome.

You now understand the complexity of diagnosing IBS. But let's assume that you are an expert in your field (you are getting closer), and you are very accurate in your ability to diagnose IBS. The next question is, "How do you treat IBS." What is the best form of treatment? Well, you are about to find out. Is it changing your diet, or taking medication, or is some ancient exotic natural formula the best treatment? Let's look at a number of studies that researchers have completed that will give you more information about what treatments are best in helping you with your IBS symptoms.

11

WHAT ARE THE CURRENT STRATEGIES FOR TREATING IBS?

You have learned that the criteria for diagnosing IBS continue to change and evolve. It only stands to reason that because no cure has been found for Irritable Bowel Syndrome, that many forms of therapy have become available to treat the symptoms, and of course some treatments are more effective than others.

More and more, complementary and alternative medicine (CAM) practices are being used for treatment. Some of the other options that are used in the treatment of IBS are acupuncture, biofeedback, traditional Chinese medicine, cognitive behavior therapy (CBT), reflexology, relaxation training, stress management, the use of audio recordings, and of course hypnosis (hypnotherapy).

At the present time, there is not enough evidence to support the use of Traditional Chinese medicine (TCM), particularly acupuncture, or meditation, or reflexology for treatment of IBS. Let's take a look at some of the CAM treatments that have been evaluated for IBS therapy.

CAM practices can be arranged into the following groups: manipulative and body-based practices, mind-body practices, and natural products. Natural products include herbal medicines, minerals, peppermint oil, prebiotics, prebiotics, and vitamins. Exclusion diets, even though they avoid rather than add certain foods, fall into the natural products group. Mind-body practices include CBT, hypnosis, meditation, and relaxation. These practices use the mind to affect physical functioning. Manipulative and body-based practices include chiropractic, massage, and reflexology. Traditional Chinese medicine (TCM) includes both acupuncture and herbal medicine. Acupuncture is considered a combination of energy-healing therapy, manipulative and body-based practice, and mind-body medicine.

Acupuncture

Acupuncture has been used in China for thousands of years. It involves the use of sharp, thin needles inserted into the body at "acupuncture points." Acupuncture is based on the theory that energy (Qi) moves through channels (meridians) in the body. The smooth flow of energy is regulated by activating specific locations on these meridians with the use of acupuncture needles.

The World Health Organization has stated that acupuncture is an effective treatment for over forty medical problems. Some of these include allergies, childhood illnesses, disorders of the eyes, nose and throat, GI tract disorders, gynecological problems, nervous conditions, and respiratory conditions. Acupuncture has been used in the treatment of alcoholism and substance abuse, and has been shown to be effective for treating arthritis, chronic pain, headaches, pregnancy, and motion sickness. It has also been used to reduce the negative symptoms of invasive Western treatments like chemotherapy and nausea due to surgery.

Acupuncture is considered most effective as a preventive treatment, or before a health condition becomes acute; however, it has also been used to help patients suffering from cancer and AIDS.

Unfortunately, the therapeutic value of acupuncture in IBS treatment is unclear. Many small studies reported that acupuncture did improve bowel symptoms and at the same time, increased the threshold of rectal pain; however, these findings were not supported by sham-controlled studies. Even in sham-controlled studies that have used either acupuncture points with no stimulation, non-acupuncture points, or specially designed "needles," a standard blinded approach has not yet been defined.

Acupuncture like TCM shares an individualized approach (which means they are highly variable) and this approach is difficult in a clinical trial setting. Western medical evaluation requires a standardized protocol in a clinical trial setting and does not reflect real-life clinical practice. There is no agreement on exactly what "standard" points are best in the treatment of IBS. For some individuals electro-acupuncture is required and for others manual needling is used. There is also no agreement on duration or frequency of treatment. Because western medicine does not recognize an individualized approach compared to a standardized protocol, western medicine does not support the use of acupuncture for treatment of IBS.

Herbal Medicine

Herbal therapies have been widely used to treat various GI tract issues. TCM formulations have been studied the most of all herbal treatments. From a TCM perspective, IBS is a syndrome of "Liver Overacting on the Spleen." This causes symptoms such as recurrent abdominal distention, abdominal pain, and borborygmus (in TCM this is Wind in the abdomen). One formulation called Tong Xie Yao Fang functions to soothe the liver, invigorate the spleen, relieve spasm and pain, and regulate the flow of Qi and the function of the stomach. In simple terms, it eliminates painful diarrhea and the urge to go to the bathroom.

The latest studies and meta-analyses confirmed the value of herbal medicine for treating IBS; however, most studies had flawed designs and were of poor quality. Since conventional medical science does not recognize Qi, it cannot explain the effects of TCM related to such things as gut motility, hormonal function, or visceral sensation.

Also because many of the studies are done in China, the safety of herbal medicine remains a major concern. There has been a lack of accurate documentation of adverse events and safety based on accepted conventional medical standards. It is felt that impurities and contaminants, such as heavy metals, cannot be predicted or controlled in herbal formulas.

Another problem that conventional medical science has with herbal formulations is that there is a problem authenticating herb activity because in some cases formulations contain more than ten herbs. TCM typically uses an individualized approach (meaning that different individuals require variable amounts of each herb) and this approach is difficult in a clinical trial setting. Because of these and other issues, current western medical evidence does not support the effectiveness of TCM for the treatment of IBS.

In a 1998 study, done by Bensoussan et al.[1] (Bensoussan is a well-recognized researcher making progress in proving the evidence for Chinese medicine), 116 IBS patients were randomly placed into one of three groups. One group used personalized Chinese herbal formulations. The second group used a standard Chinese herbal formulation. And the third group used a placebo as a control. In this study, both the personalized Chinese herbal formulations group and the standard Chinese herbal formulation group had substantial improvement in bowel symptoms compared to the patients in the placebo group; however, 14 weeks after the completion of the study, only the personalized Chinese herbal formulations group had maintained improvement.

In 2006, a study was done by Leung et al.[2] In this study, 119 Chinese patients with predominant diarrhea (IBS-D) symptoms that fulfilled Rome II criteria were recruited, and were randomly placed into two groups. 60 IBS-D patients received standardized Chinese herbal medicine and 59 IBS-D patients received a placebo. This study did not have the same positive results as the Bensoussan study. The results of this study showed that the standardized Chinese herbal medicine group had no significant difference in symptom improvement compared to the placebo group.

Even though there is a long tradition and extensive practice of acupuncture and herbal medicine, based upon conventional clinical trial methodology, there is not enough evidence to support their therapeutic use as a treatment for IBS. Again, the main problems are related to authenticating herbal formulations and standardizing acupuncture protocols.

Reflexology

Only a small single-blind study involving 34 patients was carried out on reflexology. The patients were divided into either a reflexology foot massage group or a non-reflexology foot massage control group. No significant difference was noticed in either group related to typical IBS symptoms. Also, reflexology has not been shown to be effective for treating other diseases. Because of this, existing evidence does not endorse the use of reflexology for treatment of any medical condition.

Now let's take a more in-depth look at some of treatment methods that are sometimes used in hypnotherapy, including CBT.

Cognitive Behavioral Therapy (CBT)

Although diet and medication are conventional medicine's one-two-punch, conventional medicine does support adding CBT for the treatment of IBS (usually CBT is suggested if changes to diet, and prescribed medication have had no effect for over one year). CBT is based on the principle that the way you think (cognitive) affects how you react (behavioral), and your thinking and reactions affect how you feel (physiology). IBS patients sometimes interpret visceral sensations in a way that tends to stress them out when they occur. CBT gives patients a sense of confidence and control so they can stay positive, relax more, and respond differently to their IBS symptoms. As they do this they will typically notice a reduction in their pain levels.

In 1987, Blanchard et al.,[3] conducted the first study which included a component of CBT as a treatment for IBS. In this study 14 patients participated in a treatment program which included biofeedback, relaxation training, and stress-coping strategies.

Seven years later in 1994, the first study using only CBT for IBS was conducted again by Blanchard et al[4]. In this study 20 patients were split into either the CBT group, or a waiting list control group. The CBT group received ten sessions of individual CBT. At the three-month follow-up, 80% of the CBT group reported a significant clinical improvement, compared to the control groups 10% improvement.

There are many strategies that are used in CBT including assertiveness training, coping skills, education, and progressive muscle relaxation. Since CBT tends to have a structured format, it lowers the inconsistency between treatment studies, allowing for a more accurate analysis of the treatment. CBT is goal-oriented by nature, and typically comprises of 20 sessions or less.

In 1998, Toner et al.,[5] created the first study that used a CBT protocol specially developed for treating IBS. This study did not demonstrate any significant differences between the CBT group and the control group.

In general though, study results have shown that CBT patients improved significantly when compared with placebo, and CBT is considerably more effective than educational treatment at both lowering anxiety, and improving quality of life. Studies have also shown that CBT is more effective than conventional medical treatment (even if the medical treatments included prescription medication), and CBT has a better track record with patients who had bloating or depressive symptoms.

Typically, people with IBS also have anxiety or depression (called co-morbid psychological conditions). In fact somewhere between 54 to 94% of IBS sufferers have one or both of these co-morbid conditions and CBT is effective at treating these co-morbid psychological conditions.

There is a type of feedback loop that IBS sufferers have related to anxiety. What happens is that if they experience anxiety about their abdominal pain, then their perception of pain increases. Once they notice an increase in pain, then their anxiety increases, and the loop continues. CBT can interrupt this feedback-loop which results in a significant reduction of symptom severity.

With that said, let's look at a few studies that used CBT as a treatment for IBS.

In 1996, in a study with 45 IBS patients by Van Dulmen et al.,[6] 25 patients received CBT as part of a group, and 20 patients acted as a control group. Treatment consisted of eight 2-hour group sessions over a three month period.

Each of the CBT patients were given education about how their thoughts, emotions, and environment affected their behavior, especially related to their abdominal complaints. They were also given "homework" to change their complaint-based thoughts and behaviors by trying out new ways of thinking and behaving. During the group sessions, time was spent talking about the patient's experiences with the homework, as well as mutual acknowledgment of the problems they were having handling their pain. The CBT group also received training in progressive muscle relaxation, and later on, coping imagery exercises were added.

A Daily Abdominal Complaint Score (DAC) was used. Patients rated their abdominal pain four times daily during two weeks on a scale from 0 (no pain) to 4 (serious interfering pain).

Abdominal pain was also measured daily by patients. Four times each day, they reported just how long it had been since they experienced abdominal pain based on the last time they recorded their pain.

The patients' mean DAC scores decreased by 37% for all patients in the CBT group. Interestingly, the entire control group showed a mean increase of 22%. Daily duration, daily avoidance, and a number of successful coping strategies appeared to improve significantly more for the CBT group compared to the control group.

In the year 2000, a study was done by Heymann-Monnikes et al.,[7] with 24 IBS outpatients that used a multi-component approach. One group was given assertiveness training, IBS education, cognitive coping strategies, illness-related problem-solving, progressive muscle relaxation, as well as CBT and standard medical treatment. The other group was given standard medical treatment only. The two groups were randomly assigned for ten weekly sessions.

Results of the multi-component group were significantly better than the standard medical treatment group in both symptom reduction and general well-being. The conclusion drawn from this study is that the combination of treatments plus CBT was better than standard medical treatment alone.

It's unusual to combine so many modalities into one study because it is impossible to determine which one or which combination was creating the positive results. Let's look at a couple of studies that were done by Boyce, Gilchrist, Talley and Rose[8] in 2000 and Boyce, Talley, Balaam, Koloski, and Truman[9] in 2003 that showed different results related to CBT.

In the first study in the year 2000, eight IBS sufferers (seven female, one male) between 24 to 71 years of age monitored their symptom severity on a daily basis and they also received CBT for eight sessions. CBT appeared to reduce some symptoms but had no effect on the frequency of bowel symptoms. The good news is that five of the eight IBS patients no longer met the Rome diagnostic criteria for IBS, and both anxiety and depression was reduced.

In the second study in the year 2003, 105 IBS patients (patients with resistant IBS were not included) were randomly assigned to one of three treatment groups. This study attempted to break down the multi-component approach that Heymann-Monnikes et al., had used to determine which of the individual components were effective. In this eight week study, the first group received routine clinical care. The second group received routine clinical care with relaxation training. And the third group received routine clinical care with CBT. All IBS sufferers monitored their symptom severity on a daily basis, and all subjects reported a significant improvement in bowel symptoms, such as distress, frequency, and impairment. Their anxiety and depression improved in addition to their quality of life. Interestingly, there were no significant differences among the treatment groups. The conclusion of this study demonstrated that CBT and relaxation training were not superior to routine clinical care alone in treating IBS symptoms.

In 2003, a 12-week study by Drossman et al.,[10] randomly divided 431 patients into either a group treated with CBT or a group that was mainly given education. The education group was given material to read on functional bowel disorders, and they discussed the information and reviewed their symptom diaries with a therapist. This study showed that the CBT group responded much better to treatment (70%) compared to those patients receiving education only (30%). As a note, IBS patients with depression had the least favorable effect.

In 2004 a study was done by Gonsalkorale et al.,[11] to establish whether the consistent improvement in treating IBS with hypnotherapy was related to cognitive change. The study supported the findings shown in previous research that has continued since Whorwell's first study in 1984 (I will discuss the Whorwell study later). All studies have shown that hypnotherapy reduces IBS symptoms and improves the patient's quality of life, as well as improves their psychological well-being. The study did specifically show that symptom improvement with hypnotherapy was related to cognitive change.

Psychodynamic Therapy

Around 1983, Svedlund et al.,[12] created a brief psychodynamic therapy for the treatment of IBS. The therapy was mainly supportive and focused on both coping with stress and emotional problems. In this study, 101 IBS patients were randomized to psychodynamic therapy or to a control group. The therapy group received ten sessions. The results of the study showed a significant improvement in IBS symptoms in the therapy group compared to the control group.

In 1991, Guthrie et al.,[13] performed a study that concluded that psychodynamic therapy was successful in up to 66% of IBS patients that had not responded to standard medical therapy.

In a 2003 study performed by Creed et al.,[14] a large group of IBS patients were randomized into three groups. One group received eight sessions of psychodynamic therapy (59 patients finished the study). Another group received 20 mg daily of the (SSRI) antidepressant paroxetine (43 patients finished the study), and the third group received "treatment as usual." The results of the study showed that there were no significant differences in abdominal pain. Both the psychotherapy and SSRI group did better than the treatment as usual group at improving when health-related quality of life was measured.

Relaxation Training: What is relaxation and how can relaxation training help with the symptoms of IBS?

You probably already know (and various studies have shown) that relaxation training provides several health benefits including but not limited to: decreasing anxiety, depression, and worry, as well as managing insomnia. It has been shown to be effective in helping patients cope with life-threatening illness, managing chronic pain, and promoting general health. A British study concluded that relaxation was very successful in increasing pain tolerance and at the same time, decreasing some of the symptoms associated with chronic pain. Relaxation training is also an essential part of any stress management program.

Stress has been long thought to be a major contributing factor in the cause of IBS symptoms. It is believed that relaxation acts as a coping skill that can be used immediately when a person is stressed out, or in pain. The process of relaxation also prevents some of the harmful effects of stress. Relaxation techniques, when used on a regular basis, can improve the immune system and has been linked with an improved survival rate of cancer patients.

In 1993, an eight week study by Blanchard et al.,[15] was done using 16 IBS patients who were divided equally into two groups. One group received more than ten sessions of muscle relaxation training, and they were required to practice at home. The other acted as a control group and only monitored their symptoms. In both groups, patients kept a daily diary of the severity of seven symptoms. The seven symptoms monitored were abdominal pain, abdominal tenderness, bloating, constipation, diarrhea, flatulence, and nausea. The daily diaries were collected for four weeks before the start of the study to use as a baseline and again collected four weeks after the study for comparison. 50% of the muscle relaxation group showed clinical improvement at the end of treatment compared to controls.

In 2001, a study by Keefer and Blanchard[16] was done that tested the effectiveness of another type of relaxation that was created by Herbert Benson in 1975. This relaxation technique is called relaxation response meditation (RRM). Meditation is frequently used to treat a range of psychological and pain disorders including anxiety, depression, cancer pain, fibromyalgia, headache, and lower back pain.

This study used 13 participants, and was designed to compare RRM plus symptom monitoring, with symptom monitoring alone. For additional data, the RRM group were asked to keep a record of the length of time they practiced and they were also to rate their level of relaxation before and after each practice.

67% of the RRM group had clinically improved compared to the symptom monitoring only group in the reduction of belching, bloating, constipation, diarrhea, and flatulence.

To gather even more information, six weeks after starting the study, the symptom monitoring only group was added back into the RRM plus symptom monitoring group and they received six weeks of treatment.

The "new" group significantly improved (86% clinically improved), suggesting that the improvement was due to the RRM training.

A one-year follow-up of this study showed that RRM training had caused significant reductions in abdominal pain, bloating, diarrhea, and flatulence.

So it appears that some type of relaxation training will reduce your IBS symptoms. You might be asking yourself, what are the different types of relaxation techniques, and which method might be best for me? Since there are subtle differences produced by various methods of relaxation, you should choose a relaxation technique that works best for you.

The ability to relax is developed through practice. Research indicates that at least four sessions are critical for a person to show any lasting benefit from relaxation training. Regular practice of relaxation appears to be critical in learning how to become deeply relaxed and benefits continue to increase over the first ten relaxation sessions. Here are four relaxation techniques that you might want to investigate.

Relaxation Technique 1: Meditation

The relaxation technique known as meditation originated in India over 3,000 years ago. There are many different types of meditation, but the most common types are breath meditation, mindfulness meditation, and transcendental meditation. Each form of meditation requires being in a quiet place, sitting in a comfortable position, and focusing your attention on something specific. In breath meditation, you focus your attention on your breathing … breathing in and out … breathing in and out. In mindfulness meditation, your attention centers on thoughts that enter the mind. And in transcendental meditation, your attention is focused on a word or sound.

Relaxation Technique 2: Progressive muscle relaxation

Active progressive muscle relaxation focuses your attention on feeling the differences between tensing and relaxing muscles. So it involves tensing and relaxing the major muscle groups of the body while breathing slowly and deeply. Some progressive muscle techniques start at the top of the head and work downwards, while others start at the toes and work up toward the top of the head. Whatever direction is being used, each major muscle group is tensed and then relaxed.

Relaxation Technique 3: Autogenic training

Autogenic relaxation training requires focusing on different parts of the body, and like progressive muscle relaxation, your breathing is slow and deep. In autogenic training, you imagine certain body parts are becoming warm and heavy. Interestingly, the reason that autogenic training works is not completely understood. One theory suggests that when you relax your body, you also relax the autonomic nervous system, and it's the autonomic nervous system that controls involuntary functions like blood pressure, heartbeat, and digestion.

Relaxation Technique 4: Guided imagery

Guided imagery is used a lot in hypnosis and it uses a person's imagination to create relaxing places or images. In creating the images, you want to use as many of the five senses as possible. One typical guided imagery journey is imagining lying on a beach.

"So go ahead and picture and imagine you're lying on your favorite beach. The temperature is just right, and you can hear the sound of the waves, and even children laughing off in the distance. You could be lying on the warm sand, or maybe you're just relaxing in a comfortable padded lounge

chair. You can smell the salt air, the suntan oil, and even the fragrant tropical flowers."

It turns out that a vividly visualized image has the same relaxing effect on your body as actually experiencing the situation you're thinking about. There is scientific data that supports this fact that your body cannot tell the difference between a real event and one that is vividly imagined. Kosslyn and Albert performed PET (Positive Omission Typography) studies where they viewed the areas of the brain that "lit up" when patients experienced certain events or recalled events from their memory. The PET scans showed the same parts of the brain being activated no matter if the people were actually experiencing or recalling the events, or just vividly imagining the event.[17]

The Use of Recording in Treating IBS

In the year 2000, a study was performed in which gut-directed hypnotherapy was compared with a carefully-prepared recording. This was a small randomized study of IBS patients that included 37 women and 15 men. Each of the IBS patients had not responded to either dietary or pharmacological measures.

In this small study, 76% of the hypnotherapy patients improved and 59% of the patients that only used a daily carefully-prepared hypnotic recording improved. Although the patients that used only the daily hypnotic recording had a slightly lower success rate than the direct hypnotherapist-to-patient interface, the study did show that daily use of a hypnotic recording is effective at reducing or eliminating IBS symptoms. Therefore, gut-directed hypnotherapeutic recordings are a cost effective form of treatment.

Since so many books talk about the IBS diet cure, let's look at the next chapter and briefly go over some of the studies related to diet.

You're about to learn about what you should avoid or add (if anything) to your diet.

12

CAN CHANGES IN DIET
REDUCE IBS SYMPTOMS?

*"A dietary approach to the Irritable Bowel
Syndrome has not, in the majority of
cases, solved the patient's discomfort ..."*

*- Henry Janowitz, M.D.,
Gastroenterologist Emeritus,
Mount Sinai School of Medicine*

You now know that there have been studies on alternative methods
of treating IBS. The methods that you need to focus on are CBT,
relaxation training, stress management, the use of audio recordings,
and of course as you will learn later, hypnosis. The next method
that we will be looking at is diet. Can changing your diet help
reduce your IBS symptoms?

The conventional medical treatment for IBS has been two-fold, that
is, changes to the patient's diet, and over the counter drugs as well
as prescription drugs. Remember that roughly 25%[1] of people that
have IBS are helped by diet and medication, so careful eating for
these people will reduce IBS symptoms. The goal with diet
modifications is to find and exclude "trigger foods" to reduce
symptoms.

If you have been diagnosed with IBS, then it's a good idea to keep a
journal noting the foods that seem to cause distress that you can
discuss with your doctor. The food journal should include things
like the type of food consumed, type of symptoms (if any) after
eating food, and the quality and frequency of bowel movements.

The most common trigger foods for IBS patients are foods with high fat content, and spicy foods. Reducing trigger foods will provide temporary relief, but diet adjustment seldom leads to long-term improvements. Besides spicy foods and foods with a high fat content, the following is a list of foods that **may** trigger IBS symptoms that you should pay more attention to when completing your food journal:

Alcohol

Artificial sweeteners

Butter

Caffeine

Carbonated beverages

Chocolate

Coconut milk

Coffee

Citrus juices

Dairy products

Egg yolks

Fried foods

Oils

Processed foods

Red meat

Refined sugar

Vitamin and mineral supplements may also cause GI troubles for people with IBS. Vitamin C can cause abdominal cramps, diarrhea and gas. Calcium and iron sometimes has a constipating effect, while magnesium may act like a laxative.

Diet Control and Elimination Diet

IBS patients often report that intolerance to certain foods precedes symptoms, so it is natural for them to ask for dietary advice. They may want to consult a registered dietitian to help them make changes to their diet. Dietary exclusion is a common practice, and it is sometimes suggested that dairy products be excluded from their diet, because this may be the sole cause of their symptoms. Wheat (gluten), caffeine-containing products such as chocolate, cocoa, coffee, tea, and many fizzy drinks (especially colas) are foods (and drinks) that frequently can cause symptoms.

Recently, foods shown to have IgG titers, such as beef, lamb, pork, and wheat (IgG4 antibodies have been associated with food-hypersensitivity, and titers are a way of expressing concentration) were found to cause symptoms. Foods high in IgG4 titers were excluded from the diet of 25 IBS patients for 6 months. Substantial improvements were observed in bowel movements, pain, and quality of life.

In another study, 150 IBS patients were broken into two groups for three months. One group had a diet excluding all foods associated with raised IgG antibodies, and the other group acted as a control. The results of this study showed that excluding all foods associated with raised IgG antibodies resulted in a significant reduction in symptom score, especially among patients with high compliance.

Besides having a problem with compliance, the problem with using an exclusion diet for IBS is that as you might expect, it impairs a person's quality of life. Relaxation of the diet by eating foods that raise IgG antibodies often leads to a recurrence of symptoms.

Alcohol

For some people, alcohol may trigger symptoms including cramping and diarrhea. Alcohol has also been known to disrupt sleep, which further contributes to an imbalance and disturbance of bodily functions.

Antibiotics

Antibiotics are not indicated for long-term use even though they are sometimes used as a treatment for refractory diarrhea. Antibiotics change bowel flora, and researchers have found that abdominal symptoms in people that have taken antibiotics occur about three times more often than controls. Bowel symptoms may occur four months later which makes it difficult to rule out other problems, such as trigger foods.

Caffeine

Caffeine can contribute to abdominal cramping and diarrhea. Caffeine can also aggravate anxiety, which we know can contribute to digestive tract symptoms.

Fat

Fat, especially saturated fat, trigger stomach cramps and the sudden need to have a bowel movement, because fats promote contractions. Fats may also trigger bloating and distention.

Fiber

It is a commonly held belief that dietary fiber may lessen IBS symptoms, especially constipation; however, it has a limited effect on decreasing diarrhea or reducing pain. Fiber has a number of properties that should reduce constipation by providing lubrication, and bulking the stool by having the stool retain water. The goal of enough dietary fiber is to produce soft, painless bowel movements. Additional fiber in a diet accelerates the transit time in the GI tract, produces bulkier and softer stools, while easing defecation and promoting peristalsis. Breads, cereals, fruits, vegetables, and whole grains are good sources of fiber. High-fiber diets gently distend the colon and this may help prevent spasms. Unfortunately, high-fiber diets may cause bloating and gas, which if you're lucky, may go away within a few weeks of discontinuing a high-fiber diet.

In 2006, a study of 100 consecutive primary-care (see note) IBS patients (Miller, Lea, Agrawal and Whorwell[2]), were asked to fill out a self-report questionnaire based on their consumption of bran and how bran affected their symptoms. Primary-care patients saw a 27% improvement in their symptoms. Secondary-care (see note) patients saw a 10% improvement. Symptoms were exacerbated in 22% of primary-care patients and 55% of secondary-care patients. 51% of primary-care and 33% of secondary-care patients reported that bran had no effect on their symptoms. Of the 100 participants, 48 had previously tried one or more commercial fiber products. In this group the results were about the same with 25% reporting an improvement, 19% reporting a worsening, and 56% reporting no change.

Note: Primary-care generally consists of basic health care, such as treatment of colds, flu, and simple diagnostic procedures. It can also include some preventative care and education.

Secondary Care includes more complicated treatments and procedures. It includes general surgery, and internal medicine, occupational therapy, physiotherapy, speech therapy, etc.

In 1994, another study of 100 IBS sufferers (all of which had tried bran) was conducted on the effects of bran consumption (Francis and Whorwell[3]). In this study, 55% reported worsening of symptoms, and only 10% reported an improvement. Bran exacerbated all symptoms of IBS, with bowel disturbance most often negatively affected, followed by abdominal distension and abdominal pain. The results of this study strongly suggest that using bran for IBS patients should be reconsidered.

Guar gum

Guar gum is a thick, gluey substance produced by nearly all plants and some microorganisms. It is a soluble fiber that is used as a thickener and an emulsion stabilizer in food processing. Soluble fiber promotes bacterial growth in the colon, and hydrolyzes the stool as well. Guar gum is routinely used in products such as cheese, ice cream, and processed cold meat. Partially Hydrolyzed Guar gum (PHGG) reduces gas production, which causes a reduction in bloating.

Because it reduces constipation, PHGG can be used for the treatment of IBS-C, and it is also effective in the treatment of patients suffering from IBS-D.

Peppermint oil

Peppermint oil is a naturally occurring oil taken from the leaves and flowering tops of the peppermint plant. Recent studies have shown that it may be a trouble-free and useful treatment for IBS patients. It has antispasmodic qualities that relax GI smooth muscles, and is commercially available in an enteric-coated preparation for treatment of IBS. Peppermint oil must be taken in the form of an enteric-coated capsule because if it is released in the stomach (for example if the patient chews the capsule), then this may lead to heartburn because the esophageal sphincter will relax and then stomach acid backs up into the esophagus.

In 1997, 110 IBS patients (66 men and 44 women; 18-70 years of age) were divided into two groups taking either the enteric-coated peppermint oil Colpermin, or a placebo (Liu et al.[4]). Results showed that the peppermint oil group did better than the placebo group. Abdominal pain reduction was 79% (29 patients were pain-free) compared to 43% (4 were pain-free) of the placebo group. Abdominal distension reduction was 83% compared to 29%. Reduced stool frequency was 83% compared to 32%. Reduced borborygmus was 73% compared to 31%, and flatulence was reduced by 79% compared to 22%. Similar results have occurred in studies with children with a 75% reduction in abdominal pain

The major advantage of peppermint oil is its safety profile (however, the safety of peppermint oil during pregnancy is not clear). The common side effect of heartburn is easily preventable if patients use enteric-coated capsules and they do not chew the capsules.

Prebiotics

Our GI tract contains a complicated population of bacteria known as microbiota. Through exchanges with nutrients and the gut, these bacteria adjust GI functions that may be beneficial to the host. Recently, altered colonic microbiota has been implicated in many gastrointestinal diseases, and studies suggest that the composition of colonic microbiota is disturbed and unstable in IBS patients.

Prebiotics were first identified and named by Marcel Roberfroid in 1995. Roberfroid's definition in the 2007 *Journal of Nutrition* was as follows:

> "A prebiotic is a selectively fermented ingredient that allows specific changes, both in the composition and/or activity in the gastrointestinal microflora that confers benefits upon host well-being and health"

Most prebiotics are carbohydrates such as fructose, galactose, and lactulose and may be found in Jerusalem artichokes, soybeans, unrefined barley, and unrefined wheat. Prebiotic oligosaccharides are marketed in tablet form and may be added to processed foods.

Galactooligosaccharide has been shown to selectively stimulate gut bifidobacteria in IBS patients and is effective for alleviating symptoms.

Probiotics

The root of the word *probiotic* comes from the Greek word *pro*, meaning "promoting" and *biotic*, meaning "life." The World Health Organization and the Food Agricultural Organization of the United Nations define probiotics as, "live micro-organisms which when administered in adequate amounts confer a health benefit on the host."

Probiotics are natural therapeutic agents and produce a first line defense against the colonization of pathogenic organisms. The normal microbial gut population consists of anaerobes including Bifidobacterium, Clostridium, Lactobacillus, Peptococcus, and many others. They have been shown to enhance gut barrier function, inhibit pathogen binding, and reduce mucosal permeability.

The therapeutic benefit of probiotics in the treatment of IBS has been evaluated by a number of randomized placebo-controlled trials using certain species of Lactobacillus and Bifidobacterium. In a 2005 trial consisting of 77 patients, two probiotics were compared against placebo. The patients given Lactobacillus showed no significant change when compared with placebo; however, the group who received Bifidobacterium made considerable improvement with regard to abdominal pain/discomfort, bloating/distension and bowel movement. Studies about the benefit of probiotics are also confirmed in meta-analyses. Probiotics have been shown to improve IBS symptoms and quality of life. To date, the most advantageous delivery mode of probiotics to the colon remains undetermined.

Wheat

Some people have a wheat intolerance that triggers symptoms of abdominal distention, bloating, cramping, diarrhea, or gas. Wheat is found in most breads, crackers, pasta, as well as in many other foods.

Some people also have gluten sensitivity, which is actually a specific sensitivity to the gluten component of wheat. Celiac disease is an important condition to rule out for diagnosing IBS, particularly if the patient is showing signs of diarrhea or weight loss.

Since diet and medications are the usually standard medical treatment, I guess to be complete, pharmacological solutions should be investigated. Let's take a look at some of the studies that have already been done.

13

DO PHARMACOLOGICAL TREATMENT APPROACHES WORK?

Your education now includes diet, and you know that foods with high fat content and spicy foods can cause problems. For most IBS sufferers, diet adjustment seldom leads to long-term improvements. You have learned that adding fiber to your diet typically causes more problems than it solves, but Guar gum, Peppermint oil, and the probiotic Bifidobacterium help reduce symptoms.

If you're looking for that magic-bullet in the form of a pill for a treatment cure for IBS, well, you're probably going to be disappointed. Medications are a part of the conventional "diet and medication" protocol currently used in relieving IBS symptoms. It wasn't until 1999 that any medications were specifically approved for the treatment of IBS. As of this writing, there is no medication specifically used for the treatment of IBS-M, which is the largest sub-type of IBS. In general, medications have been inconsistent and unsatisfactory, which means that the majority of patients experience little or no long-term relief.

Let's look at the drawing below and see what type of pharmacological treatment approaches are used for the various symptoms of IBS.

Drug Treatment Used For IBS

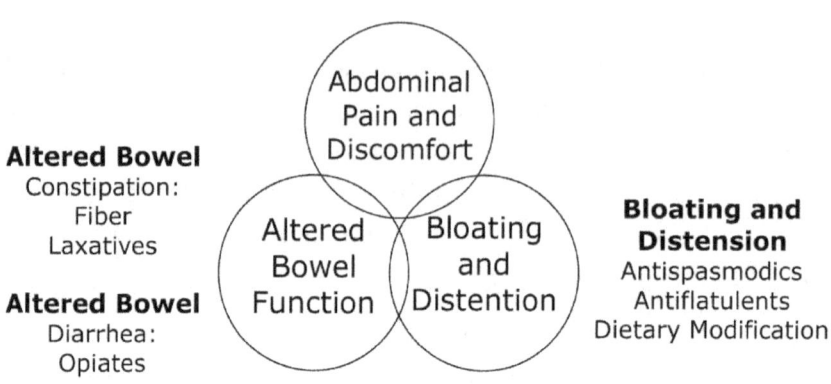

Abdominal Pain and Discomfort
Antidepressants
- TCA's / SSRIs
Antispasmodics

Altered Bowel
Constipation:
Fiber
Laxatives

Altered Bowel
Diarrhea:
Opiates

Bloating and Distension
Antispasmodics
Antiflatulents
Dietary Modification

Besides over-the-counter medications, there are a number of prescription drugs currently prescribed for IBS. In this section we'll review the use of medications in the treatment of IBS. The goal of these medications is to reduce the severity of IBS symptoms and they fall into four main categories:

1. Antispasmodics and laxatives.

2. Antidepressants and anti-anxiety medications.

3. Antidiarrheal agents.

4. Serotonergic modifying drugs.

Antispasmodics

Abdominal pain is a chief symptom in IBS and therefore the most frequently prescribed drugs for IBS are antispasmodics. Antispasmodics are motility and sensation altering medications. They are usually prescribed to help control colon muscle spasms and work to temporarily relieve discomfort from cramping because of their muscle relaxing properties. They also reduce the colon's response to eating and stress. The most commonly prescribed antispasmodic drugs are Anaspaz or Levsin (hyoscyamine), Bentyl (dicyclomine), Donnatal (belladonna/phenobarbital), and Colofac (mebeverine).

In 2005, a controlled study of 149 patients with moderate or severe Irritable Bowel Syndrome resistant to the antispasmodic Mebeverine was carried out in the UK by Kennedy et al.[1] The study compared the effectiveness of the antispasmodic Mebeverine, used in conjunction with Cognitive Behavioral Therapy (CBT), with Mebeverine used by itself. The Mebeverine/CBT group had 72 patients and 77 patients were placed in the Mebeverine only group. The Mebeverine/CBT patients had a greater symptomatic improvement and there were significant improvements as measured by the work and social adjustment scales. No group was studied to determine if it was the CBT alone that had produced these results.

There have been numerous trials evaluating the effectiveness of antispasmodic agents in the treatment of IBS. Both antispasmodics and antidepressants (see below) can worsen constipation. To date, the consensus is that antispasmodics are of questionable value.

The following is a short list of some of the antispasmodics prescribed for the treatment of IBS:

Dicyclomine (Bentyl)

Propantheline

Belladonna/Phenobarbital (Donnatal)

Hyoscyamine (Levsin, Anaspaz)

Mebeverine (Colofac)

Laxatives

ExLax or Milk of Magnesia are likely to stimulate the bowel by causing irritation of the intestinal lining and can easily lead to dependency. Nonprescription soluble fiber supplements such as Citrucel, Fibercon, Metamucil, or Psyllium may benefit IBS-C patients with mild constipation.

Antidepressants and Anti-anxiety Medications

Drugs prescribed for IBS that affect the Central Nervous System (CNS) include a large group of antidepressants and anti-anxiety medications. The effectiveness of these drugs for IBS is not well understood, but CNS drugs have both physiological and psychological effects on pain and behavior, and they may prove to be the most effective long-term medication for IBS sufferers (only time will tell).

Tricyclic antidepressants (TCAs) are recognized for relieving pain. TCAs are used in low doses to reduce abdominal pain in IBS patients. Amitriptyline, Desipramine, Doxepin, and Trimipramine, are all TCAs that have been studied in clinical trials.

In 2003, a controlled study involving 216 patients was performed comparing the use of desipramine versus placebo (Drossman et al.[2]). The original data showed that there were no noteworthy differences between desipramine (60%) and the placebo (47%). Further analysis showed that desipramine has a benefit for those patients with IBS-D. Patients with IBS-C did not improve probably because of the drying quality of the medication. Because of this study, TCAs have been used for patients suffering from IBS-D; sometimes in combination with loperamide (Imodium).

Selective Serotonin Reuptake Inhibitors (SSRI)

SSRIs such as Zoloft (sertraline), are recommended (in low-dosage) for moderate-to-severe IBS in which pain is predominant or when other therapies have failed. SSRIs are used by doctors in clinical practice for those patients with concomitant depression. SSRIs are considered to have comparatively lower side effects compared to TCAs.

Serotonin is an important neurotransmitter in the GI tract and helps control the regulation of motor and sensory functions. IBS patients often have comorbid psychiatric diagnoses (such as anxiety, depression, and sleep disorders), and SSRIs serotonin and noradrenaline reuptake inhibitors (SNRIs) may be useful if the patient has any of these conditions.

Some SSRIs (Paxil, Celexa, Prozac, and Zoloft), have been shown to trigger severe IBS attacks in diarrhea-predominant patients (IBS-D).

In 2006, a six week controlled study involving 23 (non-depressed) IBS patients was performed comparing SSRI Citalopram versus placebo. Any patients with a primary depressive disorder were disqualified from this study. Even though Citalopram had no effect on changes in mood, rectal distension or stool pattern, it was better than placebo in reducing abdominal pain, bloating, and the impact symptoms have on daily life (Tack et al.[3]).

The following is a short list of some of the antidepressants prescribed for the treatment of IBS:

Amitriptyline (Elavil)

Sertraline (Zoloft)

Paroxetine (Aropax)

Desipramine (Norpramin)

Clomipramine (Anafranil)

Doxepin (Sinequan)

Trimipramine (Surmontil)

Antidiarrheal Medication

Loperamide (Imodium) and diphenoxylate (Lomotil) are the medications of choice for patients suffering from diarrhea, but do not affect pain. They reduce diarrhea symptoms by slowing GI transit time, thus increasing the absorption of water and Loperamide also decreases urgency. A number of studies have shown that Loperamide is effective for patients suffering from diarrhea (IBS-D), especially those who have no abdominal pain.

Serotonergic Modifying Drugs

Lotronex (alosetron hydrochloride) is a 5-hydroxytrytamine receptor (5-HT3) antagonist and is helpful in treating women suffering from IBS-D. Studies indicate that Lotronex lessens diarrhea and also reduces abdominal pain and urgency.

Lotronex has been reapproved with **significant restrictions** by the U.S. Food and Drug Administration (it is not available in the UK) and doctors have been advised to prescribe this drug only after conventional therapy has failed. Patients taking Lotronex should be aware that it can have serious side effects such as severe constipation or decreased blood flow to the colon.

In female patients suffering from IBS-C who have failed to respond to standard laxatives, Zelnorm (Tegaserod) is a 5-HT3 agonist that used to be prescribed. Tegaserod is used in numerous countries; however, it too is not available in the UK, and as of 2007 is no longer available in the US. Zelnorm had been approved in the US for the short-term (4 to 6 weeks) treatment for women with IBS-C. The drug accelerates GI transit time, increases fecal water and intestinal secretion, and reduces visceral hypersensitivity.

In double-blind placebo-controlled studies (one study in 2001, and two studies in 2002) the use of Zelnorm was compared with placebo in patients suffering from IBS-C. The results showed a statistical difference between Zelnorm compared to placebo. Not only did constipation and abdominal pain get better, but in the 2002 studies that used 6 mg twice daily over a 12 week period, a noticeable different in bloating, frequency and stool consistency was found.

Again, since the 2001 and 2002 trials, the US Food and Drug Administration decided to withdraw Zelnorm (in 2007) contending that the drug was linked to heart attack or stroke.

It is always important to follow your doctor's instructions when using any medication, even over-the-counter medications such as laxatives and fiber supplements. A worsening in abdominal bloating and gas from increased fiber intake has been reported, and if used too often, laxatives can be habit forming. As discussed before there is no one cure and no one medication (or even combination of medications) they will work for everyone with IBS.

The following is a short list of some of the serotonergic modifying drugs prescribed for the treatment of IBS:

Tegaserod (Zelnorm) (5-HT4 agonist) – with caution

Alosetron (Lotronex) (5-HT3 antagonist): For female IBS-D patients

Mosapride (5-HT4 agonist, 5-HT3 antagonist)

Renzapride (5-HT4 agonist, 5-HT3 antagonist)

Lubiprostone (Amitiza) (chloride channel activator)

Methylnaltrezone (opioid receptor agent)

Alvimopan (opioid receptor agent)

If you have IBS then you'll probably like to know how your digestive system works. So let's follow a mouth-watering cheeseburger on a trip from top to bottom, as though it's on a roller-coaster ride and see where it goes.

14

INTRODUCTION TO YOUR DIGESTIVE SYSTEM

Now that you have "diet and medication" firmly under your belt, you'll want to know more about the workings of the GI tract. I've just signed you up for your next course ... next stop, the digestive system.

Your digestive system consists of a bunch of hollow passageways that begin at your mouth and end at your anus. These systems are aided by a couple of friends, the liver, gallbladder, and the pancreas, with a few cameos from the brain and nerves. These passageways, organs, friends, and cameos get together and turn the food you eat into the energy your body needs. The digestive system both chemically and mechanically breaks down food to extract the nutrients. After the nutrients are extracted, what is left is ejected as waste products in the form of urine and feces.

Let's take an in-depth look at how a cheeseburger moves along the 30-foot journey (most of the journey is through the intestines) through the digestive system from top to bottom.

Even though the mouth is the beginning of the digestive tract, the first thing that happens when you pick up that big, juicy, cheeseburger, even before you take a bite, is that your nose smells it (and if you're into cheeseburgers, especially at Maui's *Cheeseburgers in Paradise* then you know what I mean). The brain is then sent a message that basically says that it's time to salivate, so the brain tells the nerves controlling your mouth's three salivary glands (parotid, sublingual and submandibular) to start secreting juices ... juices that make your mouth water. These three salivary glands produce between one to three pints (about 0.5 to 1.5 liters) of saliva a day.

OK, at this point you can't take it anymore, so what do you do? Well of course you bite into your mouth-watering cheeseburger. Chewing that delicious, juicy bite of cheeseburger begins to mechanically break down the cheeseburger. Because you've had that mouth-watering cheeseburger before, your salivary glands get even more excited and flood your mouth with saliva. Before that first bite leaves your mouth, an enzyme in your salivary glands called amylase begins to chemically break down the carbohydrates in the bread, which makes the cheeseburger moister and easier to swallow. The salivary glands also produce the digestive enzyme lipase which breaks down fats. This soft, moist, rounded mass is called a bolus. Once swallowing is set in motion, it becomes involuntary and continues under the control of the nerves.

At this point a decision must be made because there appears to be a fork in the road up-ahead. The corridor that we don't want to take leads to the trachea (which leads to the lungs). Unfortunately sometimes food gets a little adventurous and takes a detour down the "wrong pipe." This can occur when you're laughing or even when you're just breathing when you swallow.

The corridor that we do want to take leads to the esophagus. The esophagus is a muscular tube stretching from the pharynx to the stomach. Once you swallow and the bolus makes it into the esophagus, that first bite "slides" down your throat and into the stomach. It's actually involuntary muscle contractions (called peristalses) that cause the food to "slide" toward the stomach. Muscles in the wall of your esophagus create synchronized waves that move the bite of cheeseburger into your stomach. These muscles contract behind the bolus, pressing it ahead, while at the same time muscles ahead of it relax. This allows the food to advance without resistance.

The esophagus has a warm environment that assists in the additional break down of food. The act of swallowing closes a valve over the trachea called the epiglottis. This happens so that mouth-watering piece of cheeseburger slides into the esophagus through the upper esophageal sphincter. This sphincter is a ring-shaped muscle that opens only when food is swallowed.

There is another muscle at the end of the esophagus called the lower esophageal sphincter that lets the food into the stomach. As food approaches, pressure from the food signals what we'll call the gatekeeper, to open a ring-like muscular value. The gatekeeper prevents food from escaping back into the esophagus. If you've ever had heartburn it's because this sphincter isn't working properly and stomach acid is making its way back into the esophagus. If this happens more than just occasionally, then you might have Gastroesophageal Reflux Disease, or GERD (see diseases from top to bottom).

After moving through the esophagus portion, that first bite of delicious food finally reaches the stomach. The stomach is a sac-like organ with strong muscular walls. Think of these muscular walls like a grinder. These powerful muscles begin churning and grinding the food into smaller and smaller pieces and at the same time, glands in the stomach act as a mixer. The glands secrete hydrochloric acid and other important enzymes that continue the process of breaking down the food. The stomach also has a mucous lining that coats and protects it from its own acids. About every 20 seconds or so, the stomach's muscles contract which stirs up the acid and enzymes and turns your cheeseburger into a thick, creamy fluid called chyme. From there the food moves to the small intestine.

Some foods just can't be quickly reduced to chyme and are processed in the stomach for more than an hour. Typically, the process takes only about 20 minutes to complete. As muscle contractions continue moving chyme downward, the gatekeeper is notified to open a different valve, the pyloric valve. This valve releases a small amount of chyme (about four cubic centimeters) into the small intestine. The rest continues mixing in the stomach until the gatekeeper is once again notified to open the pyloric valve.

The small intestine is made up of three segments, the duodenum, jejunum, and ileum. The duodenum (which is the first section of the small intestine) is mainly responsible for continuing the process of breaking down food. The jejunum and ileum (the second and third section) are responsible for absorbing nutrients into the bloodstream. These three sections form a long loosely coiled tube (about 20 feet in length). Intestinal villi along the walls of the tube create a very large surface area that helps with the absorption of nutrients. During the time that food is in the small intestine, the extraction of nutrients occurs with the help of a couple of friends.

The liver has many functions (more than 500), but it's the main organ involved in digestion. The liver makes and secretes bile, which helps digest fats and eliminate waste products from the blood. The bile acids dissolve the fat, and after the fat is dissolved, it is digested by enzymes from the pancreas.

The liver's extra bile travels to the gallbladder through a channel called the cystic duct where it is stored. When food approaches the small intestines, a signal tells the gallbladder to send bile to the small intestine. If a person has had their gallbladder removed, then the liver stores extra bile in newly expanded bile ducts.

One of the things that the pancreas does is produce pancreatic juices, which are made up of digestive enzymes that assist in breaking down carbohydrates, fats, and proteins. Another thing that it does is it makes the enzyme to stimulate the liver into producing bile. It also neutralizes the hydrochloric acid from the stomach. And finally the pancreas produces the hormones glucagon and insulin, which help regulate your blood sugar levels. What is left of the bite that you took out of your mouth-watering cheeseburger is passed to the large intestine.

The large intestine is another long muscular tube (about five to six feet in length). It absorbs water and some electrolytes to produce the solid waste we know as feces. If too much water is absorbed constipation will occur, and if too little water is absorbed diarrhea will occur.

The large intestine is made up of three parts: the cecum, the colon, and the rectum. The cecum is a pouch at the beginning of the large intestine. The appendix resides in the cecum, but the appendix appears to no longer be useful in the digestive process. The colon has three parts: the ascending (right) colon, transverse (across) colon and descending (left) colon. In the ascending and transverse sections, fluids and salts are absorbed. The descending colon holds the resulting waste. Billions of bacteria that normally live in the colon help to digest the remaining food products.

The colon moves waste using peristalses; however, unlike the stomach and small intestines whose movements take a matter of hours, the waste moves very slowly (about 1 centimeter per hour) so it normally takes about a day or two for waste to get through the colon. Once the descending colon becomes full, it empties its contents into the rectum to begin the process of removing the waste from the body.

The rectum is an eight-inch chamber that connects the colon to the anus. It is where waste (feces) is stored until it leaves the digestive system through the anus as a bowel movement. As the rectal walls are stretched, a message is sent to the brain. The brain then decides if there is a need for a bowel movement, and if there is, a signal will be sent to the anus to relax the sphincter muscles.

The anus is the last part of the digestive tract, and it consists of two anal sphincters, and pelvic floor muscles. Because of the angle that the pelvic floor muscles form between the rectum and the anus, stool is kept in check by the involuntary action of the internal anal sphincter. It is in a state of continuous maximal contraction, which keeps us from going to the bathroom when we are asleep, or anytime we are unaware of the presence of stool. When we get that message that it's time to go to the bathroom, we rely on our external anal sphincter to keep the stool in until we can get to the toilet.

"Normal" bowel patterns for people (at least in the US) range from three bowel movements per day to three per week. The normal amount of stool passed in a 24-hour period would not quite fill an eight ounce glass.

We have followed that cheeseburger from one end to the other, but just eating that cheeseburger can cause a couple of problems. What happens if it's so good that you "gulp" it down? Or what if it wasn't prepared right, then what happens? Let's continue looking at some of the problems that eating that mouth-watering cheeseburger can cause.

15

DIGESTIVE PROBLEMS
FROM ONE END TO THE OTHER

Next I'll be covering the digestive problems that occur from the throat to the stomach.

Belching

Belching (or burping) is the product of air in your system. Drinking carbonated beverages or swallowing air when eating (gulping down your food), causes air to collect in the stomach. This air gets pushed back up your esophagus and then out of your mouth. Typically, three to four burps after a meal is considered normal.

GERD

Gastro-Esophageal Reflux Disease, which is also called acid reflux or heartburn, is a chronic digestive disorder. It is a condition where stomach acid regurgitates (backs up, or refluxes) into the esophagus. Once it begins, it usually is life-long and it is caused by having a "lazy" esophageal sphincter. The esophageal sphincter is the valve that connects the stomach and the esophagus. This "lazy" valve permits stomach acid to come back up into the esophagus that results in a burning sensation in the middle of the chest, which we know as heartburn.

This condition can be exacerbated if food is eaten quickly or if the person is under stress. More acid can get into the esophagus if a person is smoking (nicotine) or drinking alcohol because this seems to relax the esophageal sphincter.

Interestingly, acid reflux occurs in most individuals. In patients with GERD, the problem is either excessive acid, or the reflux happens more often, or the acid remains in the esophagus longer.

Peptic Ulcers

A peptic ulcer was originally thought to be caused as a reaction to stress. It is basically a hole in the lining of the stomach or the first part of the small intestine. It is now known that instead of being caused by stress, a peptic ulcer is caused by an invasion of the Helicobacter pylori bacterium. It can also be caused by certain medications like anti-inflammatory drugs. Whether it is bacterium or drugs, the protective mucous in the stomach is weakened and allows acid to eat through it causing a hole in the lining.

Vomiting

Vomiting (medically known as emesis) is a symptom of an underlying illness and is not a specific disease. Vomiting is the act of forcible expulsion of stomach contents up through the esophagus and mouth. Vomiting can be caused by a wide variety of conditions and one of the most common is bacteria on your food. Bacteria irritating your GI tract signal the brain and vomiting occurs. Other reasons for vomiting are overeating, or food allergies, such as lactose intolerance (see below).

Digestive Disorders from the Stomach Down

Once food passes through your stomach it enters twisting organs known as the intestines. Let's cover some of the more common disorders.

Celiac Disease

Celiac disease is an autoimmune disorder of the small intestine. People with Celiac disease experience abdominal bloating, chronic constipation, diarrhea, pain, and exhaustion. These symptoms may make you think that you have IBS. However, Celiac disease is caused by a reaction to gluten, a protein found in wheat, rye, barley, and the many foods made with these products. People with Celiac disease can't easily digest nutrients from gluten-filled foods, which can also cause vitamin deficiencies. Problems can be avoided if diets are kept gluten-free.

Constipation

For this section, let's define constipation as hard, irregular or incomplete bowel movements. "Irregular" is different for everyone, but you know what is regular for you. If your bowel movements are a normal consistency and pass without discomfort, then you're not constipated. Constipation is caused when stool stays in the large intestine for too long. Too much water is removed from the stool making it hard and difficult to pass.

From a medical standpoint, constipation is defined as less than three bowel movements per week, and severe constipation is defined as less than one bowel movement per week. Constipation also requires an immediate evaluation if it is accompanied by abdominal pain and cramps, nausea, rectal bleeding, vomiting, or weight loss.

Crohns Disease (CD)

Crohns disease is a chronic inflammatory condition that can affect any area of the GI tract, from the mouth to the anus, but it generally affects the lower part of the small intestine. It can manifest with such symptoms as abdominal cramping, diarrhea, fever, vomiting, and weight loss. Again these are symptoms very similar to IBS; however, because there is inflammation this is not IBS. When the condition is active, fruits, vegetables, and high fiber should be avoided because they tend to increase diarrhea. Also smoking cigarettes can aggravate the condition.

Diarrhea

When muscle contractions in a person's intestines happen too quickly, the intestines don't have time to absorb water from the waste matter before it is sent out of the body, and the result is diarrhea. There are many causes of diarrhea, from bacteria, to intestinal inflammation, to stress. Typically, Americans have four attacks of diarrhea each year.

Flatulence

We all know that everybody passes gas (if we're in an elevator … it wasn't me!). The average person passes gas between 10 to 25 times a day, and this is due to the breakdown of food in the large intestine. A signal is sent to the brain if excess gas is sensed in the rectum. This sounds strange, but the "brain" looks around and determines if it's a good time to release the gas. If it's OK to do so, the sphincters relax, the rectum contracts and gas is passed.

Inflammatory Bowel Disease (IBD)

IBD is a chronic inflammation that causes swelling and pain in the intestines. There are two major types of IBD: Crohns disease and ulcerative colitis. Both IBDs are auto-immune disorders that may be considered life threatening illnesses.

Lactose Intolerance

Lactose intolerance is all about the inability to digest the major sugar in milk. The milk sugar lactose is a carbohydrate that is found in dairy products and milk products. Lactose malabsorption is very common, especially in African-Americans, Asian-Americans, Hispanic Americans, and Native Americans. If your digestive system doesn't produce enough of lactase, (which is found in the small intestine), then you can't break down milk into simpler sugars that the body can digest. This intolerance is usually dose-related, which means that depending on the person, some people can tolerate small amounts of dairy products and other people cannot. People with lactose intolerance experience mild to severe bloating, cramps, diarrhea, gas, or nausea, usually within a short time after ingesting the dairy product. Notice that the symptoms are very similar to the symptoms of IBS. Usually a two week period of restricting frozen yogurt, ice cream, milk, and soft cheese, especially mozzarella and cottage cheese, is used to determine whether lactose intolerance is contributing to a person's symptoms.

Ulcerative Colitis (UC)

Ulcerative colitis causes inflammation and ulcers in the top layer of the lining of the large intestine beginning at the rectum. IBS is differentiated from UC because IBS does not have any bleeding into the bowel. The bowel is not inflamed or ulcerated, and there is no obstruction in IBS. The suggested medical treatment for ulcerated colitis is an anti-inflammatory drug such as Asocol, Rowasa, or Pentusa, and it usually takes somewhere between three to six weeks for improvement to be evident. Symptoms can manifest as anemia created by bleeding of the ulcers, large amount of mucus that is often bloody, and severe cramping. There may also be abdominal cramps, diarrhea, intestinal bleeding, and weight loss.

Good job so far. You have made it through IBS boot camp. In a short time you have read through a large amount of information so you are really up to date on your condition.

Before we move on to understanding a well-proven and clinical successful technique for reducing or eliminating the symptoms of IBS, let's do one last review. If you had been diagnosed with IBS and under your doctor's supervision for more than one year, then you would be starting from this next chapter.

16

WHAT HAVE WE
LEARNED SO FAR?

If you're an IBS sufferer that has been under your doctor's supervision for more than one year, then I want to go over a quick summary of what I think you should know about Irritable Bowel Syndrome so that I'll know that we are aware of the same information.

I'm sure by now you already know that IBS is a diagnosis of exclusion. If a patient presents with the typical ABC symptoms of IBS (A = Abdominal pain, B = Bloating, and C = Change of bowel habits), it is rare to find any other disease. Because there is no definite single cure for IBS, the current objective in IBS "treatment" is to decrease the patient's symptoms and improve their quality of life.

You now know that Irritable Bowel Syndrome is a gastrointestinal disorder characterized by abdominal discomfort or abdominal pain where there are changes in bowel movements, such as constipation, or diarrhea, or both. There is also no identifiable cause, such as an inflammation, infection or structural abnormality. There must be no pathology that can be determined for a diagnosis of IBS. It is the most common GI disorder, accounting for over 10% of primary care physicians visits, and it's estimated to take up more than 30% of a gastroenterologist's workload. To date there is no single effective standard medical treatment for IBS.

Worldwide IBS is a problem, with countries reporting 3.5% to 30% of their population having IBS. In the United States, about 20% have IBS, two-thirds of which are women.

Children as young as age nine can have IBS, and adults may display symptoms of IBS as early as age twenty. If you make it past 50 years of age then you're unlikely to ever have IBS symptoms.

Researchers cannot pin-down a single exact cause of Irritable Bowel Syndrome, probably because it will be found that there is not a single cause. Since there is no cure for IBS, many forms of treatment are available to deal with the symptoms. The conventional medical treatment for IBS originally was two-fold, that is, changes to the patient's diet and medication; however, now education is included along with suggestions for using relaxation techniques; psychotherapy is sometimes suggested if diet and medication have not worked after trying this treatment protocol for more than one year.

It is suspected that some communication between the brain and the GI tract has broken down, which leads to the symptoms of IBS. Studies have suggested that a subset of IBS sufferers have an increased awareness of sensations of the gut (visceral hypersensitivity). A patient's IBS symptoms may also be from antibiotics, gastroenteritis, genetics, or from an imbalance of neurotransmitters. Symptoms may also be from psychosocial factors or small intestine bacterial over-growth. By and large, it is accepted that emotions affect the GI tract, and it is agreed that a patient's emotional response to stress can aggravate and intensify the condition. As we continue to have a better understanding of IBS we are moving away from the old disease-based model to a bio-psycho-social model.

Studies show that IBS is more common in people with family members who have a history of GI problems, or in people who have any type of emotional, physical, or sexual abuse, or psychological conditions. Stress is also a factor in people who have IBS.

If you've had IBS for some time then I'm sure that you understand the difficulty in diagnosing IBS. You are familiar with what tests need to be run to rule out other diseases. You also realize that the criteria for diagnosing IBS are a moving target. The first accepted criteria for IBS was the Manning criteria in 1976, and then to stay up to date you had to become familiar with the Rome I (1988), Rome II (2000), and Rome III criteria (2006), knowing that as of this writing in 2014, Rome IV is on the way.

In a lot of ways the Rome III criteria made things more difficult, and yet at the same time more exacting. Sub-typing is based on stool consistency; however, IBS-C (constipation predominant) and IBS-D (diarrhea predominant) are still acceptable.

Rome III classified Functional Gastro-Intestinal Disorders into 28 categories. So IBS Doctors are now required to understand the differences between IBS, functional bloating, functional constipation, and functional diarrhea. And to make it worse, some symptoms, such as bloating, constipation, diarrhea, and pain, overlap across disorders.

IBS is specifically distinct in its definition, which is pain associated with change in bowel habit. Functional diarrhea is distinguished by loose stools and no pain. Functional bloating has no change in bowel habit.

Presuming the absence of a structural or biochemical explanation for the patient's symptoms, the Rome III diagnostic criteria for Irritable Bowel Syndrome always can be diagnosed based on at least three months of active symptoms with the onset of symptoms at least six months previously of recurrent abdominal pain or discomfort (discomfort means an uncomfortable sensation not described as pain) and also having two or more of the following:

1. Relieved with defecation; and/or

2. Onset associated with a change in frequency of stool; and/or

3. Onset associated with a change in form (appearance) of stool.

Many forms of treatment are available to care for the symptoms of IBS. Some have no effect, some help a little, and some work better than others. We know that the "typical" conventional medical treatment for IBS is done using two parts. One part changes the patient's diet, and the other part uses over-the-counter drugs as well as prescription drugs.

Complementary and alternative medicine (CAM) practices are being used more and more due to the poor outcome of just changing a person's diet and adding medications. If you are interested, I have included a chapter that is called, "What Are The Current Strategies For Treating IBS?" I've presented a brief look at some of these therapies, including acupuncture, biofeedback, traditional Chinese medicine, cognitive behavior therapy (CBT), reflexology, relaxation training, stress management, the use of audio recordings, and coming up we will take a very serious look into hypnosis and hypnotherapy.

Changes to diet (and medication) help roughly 25% of the people who have IBS symptoms. Patients often complain of diet-related symptoms[1, 2] and they have frequently tried exclusion diets with inconsistent results. Patients typically will benefit from eating small meals more often, and eating these meals slowly.

The most common trigger foods for IBS patients are foods with high fat content, and spicy foods. Reducing trigger foods will provide temporary relief, but diet adjustments seldom lead to long-term improvements.

Antibiotics may cause bowel problems four months after taking them. And although fiber (which increases gut transit time) is commonly suggested for constipation, it has been shown to exacerbate symptoms in more people than it helps.

In some IBS patients, carbohydrate malabsorption can aggravate their symptoms; however, when a study looked into the association between carbohydrate malabsorption and hypersensitivity or dysmotility, the results were negative[3].

Guar gum (which reduces gas and bloating) appears to be effective in the treatment of IBS-C, and it is also effective in the treatment of patients suffering from IBS-D.

Peppermint oil is also useful in the treatment of IBS because it has antispasmodic qualities that relax GI smooth muscles.

The jury is still out on the advantages (or disadvantages) of prebiotics, but the probiotic Bifidobacterium has shown considerable improvement with abdominal pain/discomfort, bloating/distension and bowel movement.

Medications are a part of the conventional "diet and medication" protocol, but generally, medications have been inconsistent and unsatisfactory in providing any kind of long-term relief. Remember there is no medication specifically used for the treatment of IBS-M (alternating constipation and diarrhea), which is the largest sub-type of IBS.

The goal of medications is to reduce the severity of IBS symptoms and they fall into four main categories, which are: Antispasmodics and laxatives, Antidepressants and Anti-anxiety medications, Antidiarrheal agents, and Serotonergic modifying drugs.

Today's consensus is that antispasmodics are of questionable value. Antidepressants (and anti-anxiety) medications may prove to be an effective long-term medication for IBS sufferers, but more studies need to be done to determine their value. Studies have shown that Loperamide is effective for patients suffering from IBS-D, especially those who have no abdominal pain, and studies indicate that Lotronex lessens diarrhea and also reduces abdominal pain and urgency; however, it may have serious side effects such as severe constipation or decreased blood flow to the colon.

Now that we have similar knowledge related to IBS, the question is, "Where do you go from here, and how do you get control over your IBS symptoms?" Well, get ready because:

> *"You're about to travel into another dimension, a dimension not only of sight and sound but of mind; a journey into the middle ground between light and shadow, between science and superstition. This place is on the border of man's fears and the summit of his knowledge. You're about to move into a land of both shadow and substance, of imagery, ideas, expectation, and imagination. That's the signpost up ahead - your next stop, the Hypnosis Zone!" – Adapted from the Twilight Zone opening monologue.*

Did you know that your expectations are important in resolving your IBS symptoms? It's time to use your mind, imagery, and imagination, to make the necessary changes to improve your quality of life. So open the door to the next chapter and let's see what's possible.

17

IS IT POSSIBLE TO USE IMAGERY IN HEALING?

"There is no illness of the body
apart from the mind."

- Socrates

Let's discuss how imagery can be used to help reduce or eliminate your IBS symptoms. Imagery has been present in all of the world's cultures since the earliest of times, and it is an essential healing tool of many religions. Hippocrates taught that a patient's situation as well as their emotions should be considered during their treatment. Aristotle believed that the body and soul worked together for the benefit of the individual.

Imagery is a dominant representation of the imagination. It is said that Albert Einstein imagined himself riding on a beam of light, and from this image he realized the distortion of time and space. Even Albert Einstein was quoted as saying that:

"Imagination is more important than knowledge.
Knowledge is limited. Imagination encircles the world." [1]

How we speak to ourselves does matter. Our feelings and beliefs impact every cell of our body. The mind's ability to affect the body has long been known in medicine but this ability of the mind to affect the body is really only currently accepted in the form of the placebo effect. A change in a person's symptoms as a result of receiving something that does not (directly) act on the disease is called the placebo effect. The placebo effect demonstrates that a person's belief has an effect on the outcome of their treatment. Physicians (and more recently researchers) have been studying the power of the mind for centuries. And not only is it acknowledged in medical journals but scientific methods now require a placebo to be used in drug trials (Papakostas and Daras, 2001[2]).

From the mind-body perspective, the placebo effect follows the Law of Expectancy. The Law of Expectancy states that:

> *"When someone whom you believe in or respect (such as a person of authority) expects you to perform a task or produce a certain result, you will tend to fulfill their expectation whether positive or negative."*

The first example of the Law of Expectancy that you will probably recognize most likely occurred when you were very young. Maybe you were outside playing and fell down and scraped your knee. What did you do? I'm pretty sure you ran into the house crying and your Mommy cleaned up the scrap. Maybe she even put a band-aid on it. But the most important thing she did was to kiss the "owie" and make it feel all better. She might have even said something like, "Ok, it's all better now." In this case, Mom was the person you believe in, and as a result you performed up to her expectation of feeling better.

It turns out that your expectations affect your health. How many times did you think that you were coming down with a cold or the flu, and you were saying to yourself, "I think I'm getting sick," and you probably did get sick. It's actually worse if you ask someone you trust about how you look (here comes the Law of Expectancy) and they say, "You don't look so good. Are you coming down with something?" Your brain then takes the appropriate steps to provide you with the expectancy that you are coming down with something, and this is confirmed by science.

In 2011, a study was performed by Tracey et al.,[3] on the effect of a patient's beliefs and expectations on drug efficacy. Britain and Germany researchers used functional magnetic resonance imaging (fMRI) to record how a person's feelings and past experiences can influence the effectiveness of medicines.

Researchers investigated how different expectations of 22 healthy volunteers affect the analgesic efficiency of the drug remifentanil (a potent ultra short-acting synthetic opioid painkiller).

The researchers were interested in three conditions: no expectation of analgesia, expectancy of a positive analgesic effect, and with negative expectancy of analgesia (that is, expectation of more pain).

Volunteers were asked to rate pain on a scale of 1 to 100 as heat was applied to one leg while their brains were being monitored in an fMRI scanner. The average initial pain rating as heat was applied was 66. Without the volunteer's knowledge, the researchers started giving the drug via infusion to see what effects would occur. They did this without the volunteers knowing that the drug was being administered. During this phase of the study with the same amount of heat applied the average pain rating went down to 55.

At this point the volunteers were told that the drug was now being administered, even though no change was actually made in the amount of the opioid they were receiving. After hearing that the drug was being administered, the average pain ratings dropped to 39.

Next the volunteers were then told the drug had been stopped. They were also warned that there may be an increase in pain; however, the drug continued to be given at the same dose. And what do you think occurred? Their pain intensity increased to 64. This means that their pain was almost as bad as it had been at the initial phase of the study.

The volunteers' subjective reports were validated by noteworthy changes in the neural activity in brain regions involved with the coding of pain intensity. Negative expectancy effects were associated with activity in the hippocampus, and the positive expectancy effects were associated with activity in the endogenous pain modulatory system.

The results of the study strongly suggest that the patients' beliefs and expectations affect both the therapeutic and adverse effects of any given drug. Even a powerful painkilling drug with a true biological effect can be negated if a patient believes that it will not work for them, and images of their brains show how this occurs.

The Law of Expectancy was demonstrated in the television show *MASH*. In season six, a problem arises when administering morphine to a post-op patient. The patient had an immediate adverse reaction to the morphine and it seems that the last box of morphine the 4077th had left was contaminated.

Colonel Potter discusses the options with the surgical staff. Dr. Winchester suggests using the morphine, saying that one soldier's reaction should not condemn the entire box. However, the problem is that they have a hospital full of patients and they can't risk making their patients sicker, and with no painkillers, and with no possibility of getting any more until the morning, everyone is in a tough spot.

Potter, begins telling a story that occurred when he was eight-years-old about his aunt Grace when she came down with a migraine. Ol' Dr. Schumacher (a simple country doctor) was called. He showed up, gave her a couple of pills and told her not to worry, that she would be fine and completely cured. Within a short time she was fine. Hot-lips asked what he gave her and Potter said, "It was two sugar pills." After some discussion about migraines compared to compound fractures Potter says, "The body can do remarkable things if the mind will let it." He believes that if the doctors can sell it … really sell it … that it just might work. He says if the patients believe they are being given morphine that it will work, "If it will work in their minds, it will work in their bodies."

Hawkeye and B.J. make up a batch of "special" morphine pills, and when giving the special morphine pills to the first patient Hawkeye says, "It's a very, very strong pain-killer. You'll be asleep in a few minutes." B.J. says, "These are very potent … one is more than enough." When asked how long these pills will take effect, Winchester reluctantly says, "There are a number of variable factors involved …" Hot-lips interrupts him and says, "Ten minutes solider." Everyone gives out the special morphine pills selling them as convincingly as possible.

After a short time the doctors realize that for the most part, the medication is working. Almost half of the patients are without pain, and are sleeping soundly. When one patient complains that the medication is not working, B.J. agrees to give him one more, "But that's it because these things are just too strong." Later that night, Potter points to his head and says, "The best doctor is right up here."

You might be interested to know that this episode is based on fact. During the Korean War, MASH units did run out of morphine, and when medical workers gave wounded soldiers "special" morphine pills 25 percent to 40 percent of the soldiers reported a reduction in pain. The "special" morphine pills worked because the expectation that the "medicine" would help was so strong that the patient's brains actually translated it into reality.

Let's look at an actual example of the mind's ability to affect the body that was first reported in 1957 [4], and then again in the *Psychobiology of Mind-Body Healing* [5], by Ernest Rossi in 1986. Ernest Rossi discusses a cancer patient from the 1950's named Mr. Wright.

Mr. Wright had developed a highly advanced cancer involving the lymph nodes (lymphosarcoma). All treatments had failed, and the general impression was that he was in a terminal state. Massive tumors the sizes of oranges were in his abdomen, armpits, axillas, chest, groin, and neck area. His spleen and liver were also gigantic. The staff drew one to two liters of a milky fluid from his chest every other day, and he was frequently taking oxygen by mask because the fluid was making it difficult for him to breath. Nothing could be done other than to give him sedatives to diminish any pain and discomfort he was having.

Even though the doctors had given up on him, Mr. Wright was not without faith. The reason for Mr. Wright's optimism was that he expected a new drug to come along to improve his condition. In fact, this drug had already been reported in the newspapers. The name of the experimental drug was Krebiozen.

Somehow Mr. Wright had heard that his clinic was one of a hundred places chosen by the American Medical Association (AMA) for evaluation. The AMA had decided on treating 12 cases in Mr. Wright's hospital; however, Mr. Wright was not deemed suitable because one requirement was that the patient must still be able to benefit from standard therapies. Another requirement was that the patient must have a life expectancy of a least three and if at all possible six months. Mr. Wright certainly didn't qualify for having a life expectancy of six months, and in was very unlikely that he would live more than two weeks.

When Mr. Wright heard his clinic was involved in research on Krebiozen, he pleaded to be given the Krebiozen treatments. He begged so hard for what he called his "golden opportunity," that against the rules of the Krebiozen committee, it was decided to include Mr. Wright in the test.

Injections were given three times weekly, and Mr. Wright received his first injection on a Friday and his doctor didn't see him again until Monday. His doctor actually thought that Mr. Wright might be dead by that time, and then his supply of drugs could be reallocated to another patient. When the doctor came back on Monday he was in for quite a surprise. When he'd left on Friday, Mr. Wright was having trouble breathing and was confined to his bed, but now after only one injection, he was walking around the clinic talking cheerfully with the nurses and sharing his message of happiness and joy to anyone within earshot. Immediately his doctor went to the other patients who had received their first injection on that previous Friday. There was no change in the other patients; only Mr. Wright had this dazzling improvement. His tumor masses, and I quote now, "The tumor masses had melted like snowballs on a hot stove, and in only these few days, they were half their original size!" Also, Mr. Wright had no other treatment except the single dose. As his doctor said:

"This phenomenon demanded an explanation, but not only for that, it almost insisted that we open our minds to learn rather than try to explain."

The injections were given three times weekly as intended. Much to the joy of Mr. Wright, but with much confusion and bafflement of his doctors, within ten days Mr. Wright was discharged from his deathbed. Virtually all signs of his disease had disappeared in the short time that he was given the drug, and as unbelievable as it might sound, this patient that was not long for this world, this patient that was gasping for his last breath through an oxygen mask, well this patient was not only breathing normally and full of life but he was flying his private plane at over 12,000 feet with no discomfort.

This mind-boggling situation occurred at the start of the Krebiozen trials, but within two months, inconsistent reports began to appear in the news. All of the testing clinics were describing that there were no results. Mr. Wright could be logical and scientific in his thinking, and when he heard about these reports this greatly concerned him. What was maybe more important, was that he began to lose faith in his last hope of a drug cure. As the negative reports continued to come in his health became worse, and Mr. Wright ended up back in the hospital.

Knowing something about Mr. Wright's confidence in the drug, his doctor urgently took advantage of Mr. Wright's hopefulness … just purely for scientific reasons of course. Mr. Wright's doctor came up with a further experiment to answer some of his own questions. When Mr. Wright had given up all hope on his wonder drug, his doctor decided to tell Mr. Wright a story. He told Mr. Wright to not accept what he read in the papers. He told him that the drug really shows potential, and the reason for his relapse was because the drug had a limited shelf life; and not only had that problem been corrected, but the new product was twice the strength of the original product.

The news came as a great surprise to Mr. Wright, so much so that his confidence increased, and he was eager to start again. His anticipation grew and grew with each day until the "new" drug finally arrived. His doctor then announced that a new series of injections was about to begin. The doctor, "with much fanfare and putting on quite an act," administered the first injection of this new improved Krebiozen. The doctor made a preparation, which consisted of saline and nothing more.

The results of this experiment were quite remarkable. Recovery from his second near terminal state was even more spectacular than before.

"Tumor masses melted, chest fluids vanished, and Mr. Wright became ambulatory and went back to flying again. He was the picture of health... His water injections continued since they had worked wonders and he remained symptom free for over two months."

And then the final blow occurred. The AMA announced in the press, and I quote,

"Nationwide tests show Krebiozen to be a worthless drug in the treatment of cancer."

Within a couple days of reading the report, Mr. Wright was readmitted to the hospital. With all of belief, conviction, and hope gone, he died in less than two days.

The case of Mr. Wright all too vividly illustrates the hope and the failure of our attempts at mind-body communication and healing as they currently exist. You know for example that today a person can control the growth of cancers if they can improve their immune system. It is their immune system that can destroy the cancer. Obviously Mr. Wright's immune system must have been activated by his belief in a cure. His incredibly rapid healing also suggests that his autonomic and endocrine systems must have been responsive to suggestion and enabled him to mobilize his blood system with amazing effect that must have removed the toxic fluids and waste products of his cancer. Mr. Wright's experience tells us that it was his belief in the drug Krebiozen that had mobilized the healing placebo response by activating all of his major systems of mind-body communication and healing.

So the question is, "If mind-body communication can affect severe pain like it did during the Korean War, and if mind-body communications can affect rapid healing in Mr. Wright's case, can it reduce or eliminate a person's IBS symptoms?"

At the beginning of this section, I presented that the use of imagery has ancient roots. Currently in the West, mind and body are still generally regarded as two separate entities. This is because in the seventeenth century, the holistic ancient medical beliefs related to the mind-body connection were discarded. This is primarily because of two men: Francis Bacon and Rene Descartes. Bacon maintained that science should be used to gain mastery over nature. In 1637, Rene Descartes (the French philosopher and scientist) asserted that the mind and body were separate. Descartes' stance, that later became known as the reductionist method in which **the goal was to find a single underlying biological etiology**, took over not only medical philosophy but religious philosophy as well.

From Descartes' stance, the idea of the mind playing a role in illness and disease became unimportant. Religion became associated with the spirit (or soul), and the mind was considered the seat of the soul, therefore medicine was not to tamper with it. Of course in our time, scientific studies associate the mind and body as part of a system. Any malfunction in either of them can produce illness and disease.

In the East, the mind is considered of primary importance in the treatment of disease. The mind (and especially the imagination) was (and is) used to effect changes in a person's physical, mental, and emotional states.

In ancient times, shamans were considered to have the most experience in dealing with a person's inner world, especially using expectation and imagery (the process of the imagination) to heal a person. Shamanism is, according to Achterberg[6], "the medicine of the imagination," and is ever-present throughout the world.

Around 4000 years ago, Egyptian physicians noted one could have good health by having an optimistic attitude.

Ayurveda, which is believed to be some 3,000 years old, uses sound, vibration, yoga, and imagery to improve health. Mantra yoga uses the repetition of divine names or phrases (mantras). Even though mantras can be used alone, more often than not, they are combined with other techniques including imagery. Examples of this might be to imagine a healing light or visualizing a mandala. A mandala is a geometric pattern that represents wholeness and connection between one's self and the infinite. This technique can be used in meditation or in trance induction.

Visualization is included in the healing practices in Tibetan Buddhism. Light is imagined as radiating from divinity and flowing through a person's body, filling it up and healing it both mentally and physically.

Chinese physicians noticed that periods of emotional trouble created physical illness. Chinese medicine also uses imagery to direct and redirect Qi to heal various parts of the body. In Chinese martial arts it is customary to imagine breathing in light and directing it to various parts of the body.

Sigmund Freud believed that repressed emotions resulted in physical problems. Both Freud and later Jung acknowledged the role of imagery in illness and health, particularly in dreams. Freud paid attention to mental images during dream analysis, which was the core of his psychotherapy. Jung believed that through images and symbols encountered in dreams he could get to know his patient's unconscious mind. (If you are interested in a Hawaiian Dream Interpretation process, then check out the book, *Naked Dreams: Hawaiian Dream Interpretation, 10 Steps To Uncovering The True Meaning of Dreams*[7]).

Dr. Carl Happich, who was influenced by Freud and Jung, developed a visualization technique based on Eastern meditation that offered therapeutic benefit to the individual. Happich's process began by first relaxing the body and mind through breathing exercises, after which different locations and situations were created. Happich's visualization technique activated "archetypal" images where healing could take place.

In the late 1970s, George Engel, M.D., proposed the biopsychosocial model of illness and health. Dr. Engle's model holds that multiple factors, that is, biological, which includes physical and neurochemical, psychological, which includes thoughts, attitudes, beliefs, and feelings, as well as social, which includes interpersonal relationships, are all interconnected prerequisites for health. This suggests that there are many factors that affect a patient's health. The biopsychosocial model suggests that things like the absence (or presence) of social support, biochemical abnormalities (or physical abnormalities), depression, and of course high levels of stress, can act at the cellular level to influence the state of health or illness. Our mental state and physical health are therefore unavoidably tied together.

Dr. Engel trained Douglas Grossman, M.D., a gastroenterologist from the University of North Carolina. Dr. Grossman has led the way in using the biopsychosocial model for digestive illness and health. According to Dr. Grossman:

"To have any chance of clinical success, a management strategy for Irritable Bowel Syndrome must integrate psychological, social, and biological factors, all of which influenced the path though physiology and clinical course of the disease process."

Carl and Stephanie Simonton researched the impact of using visualization techniques with their patients. Their investigation involved looking at the influence that the mind had in extending the lives of cancer patients. One study of 152 cancer patients showed that:

> *"A positive attitude toward treatment was a better predictor of response to treatment than was the severity of the disease."*

Their research (Simonton, et al., 1978[8]) found that when using relaxation and imagery techniques their cancer patients showed a 41% improvement, with 22.2% having total remission, and 19.1% tumor regression. The techniques that the Simonton's pioneered are currently a standard visualization practice in the field.

Dr. Ainslie Meares was also researching the effect of mind on disease, including that of cancer. His goal was to assist people in gaining access to the natural undisturbed calm within themselves, which he called stillness. He believed that if a state of inner stillness could be achieved, then the mind could re-activate the healing powers of the body including the immune system. Meares' therapeutic meditative approach, called the Stillness Meditation Therapy (SMT) is used today.

These are just some of the vast number of examples that have shown the power of the mind to affect the body. Other examples include the physiological effects of imagery to increase a person's heart-rate by imagining that they are running. The size of a person's pupils can be changed by simply imagining sights. Experiments have been performed demonstrating that muscle tension increases when a person imagines lifting heavy weights. And of course, GI activity can be influenced by a person's thoughts.

The results of all this research strongly suggests that physiological functions that are usually considered as involuntary may be influenced by imagery. So what is one of the best techniques that use imagery? Well, it's hypnosis. Yes I did use the "H" word ... hypnosis.

In hypnosis, suggestions are usually given in the form of imagery. And since the body is unable to tell the difference between something that is vividly imagined and "reality," then the suggested images are interpreted as "real" events. What this means for IBS sufferers is that gut-directed imagery, according to all the research, is expected to have an effect on the function of their GI tract, thus reducing or eliminating their symptoms.

If you're like most people, you have probably heard about hypnosis and at the same time you probably have many misunderstandings about it. So let's look at the next chapter and clear-up a number of the misconceptions and myths about hypnosis so that you can get the most benefit from using gut-directed imagery.

18

WHAT IS HYPNOSIS
AND HYPNOTHERAPY?

You're about to take a journey into the dimension of mind-body communication known as hypnosis. It's time to travel into the middle ground between light and shadow, between science and superstition, between fears and knowledge. You're about to move into a land of imagery, ideas, expectation, imagination, and into a place that just might finally help you significantly reduce or completely eliminate your IBS symptoms. Without any fear, it's time to investigate one of the most powerful forms of mind-body communication ... hypnosis!

Although hypnosis has become more mainstream these days, there continues to be a number of misconceptions about hypnosis. Let's face it, to the average person hypnosis appears to be absolutely magical. There is much misconception surrounding hypnosis, and yet, there is nothing supernatural about it. For most people, hypnosis is surrounded with mysticism where patients are under the control of the hypnotist. This is probably because their only exposure to hypnosis is unfortunately through stage shows or horror movies, where hypnosis is used for entertainment. Although stage hypnosis is both astonishing and real, it leaves the observer with some ideas about hypnosis that may not be quite correct. Stage shows have caused hypnosis to be made light of and have completely caused its value to be underestimated as a significant therapeutic tool.

So that you can become completely comfortable with hypnosis, let's dispel some of the misconceptions that surround it.

The number one misconception about hypnosis is that hypnosis is like sleep or a person goes to sleep while under hypnosis. This belief probably originated because many hypnotists use the word, "sleep", and because the person being hypnotized more often than not has their eyes closed and is deeply relaxed. That's where the similarities between hypnosis and sleep end. It turns out that when a person is hypnotized they are extremely attentive, aware, and focused.

Another common fear and misconception about hypnosis is that while hypnotized a person can be made to do anything. The idea of hypnosis as mind-control was popularized by the character of Svengali in George Du Maurier's novel *Trilby* (1885) and repeated over and over again by Hollywood movies ever since.

Stage hypnosis is for entertainment purposes. People are encouraged to perform amusing or bizarre or even humiliating acts (depending of course on your point of view). If hypnosis was mind-control then it would be an understandable concern. But the truth is, while hypnotized a person won't violate their own conscious moral principles, and do anything that they would not normally do in their everyday walking around state. The hypnotized person is in full control, and if a suggestion is ever given that they don't agree with, they will simply not follow the suggestion.

Dr. Milton Erickson (who I will talk about more in the next chapter) actually tested this out. Erickson was a psychiatrist and the founding president of the American Society for Clinical Hypnosis. He attempted to make his hypnotic subjects perform distasteful, disagreeable or minor criminal acts. People would perform these acts if they felt it was "just an experiment" (like you would during a stage show); however, they refused to perform the acts in situations where there might be real consequences. After performing a number of these experiments, Erickson said:

"Hypnosis cannot be misused to induce hypnotized persons to commit actual wrongful acts, against themselves or others."

Another misconception is that while under hypnosis, a person will reveal their deepest and darkest personal secrets, and of course this belief is also untrue. Hypnosis isn't a truth drug. Under hypnosis a person will only reveal what they want to reveal. They will only share something that they might consciously tell another person, such as a trusted friend or their therapist. If they have secrets that they don't want to share, then they simply won't share them. Again, you're awake and aware the entire time, so you remain in control and are free to say as much or as little as you wish.

Another misconception about hypnosis is that you won't remember what happened while you "were under." This is related to the misconception about losing control and being made to do things that you normally would not do. If for some reason a person does not remember what happened to them while under hypnosis, it's probably because they believe that they won't remember what happened to them.

There is nothing about the process of hypnosis itself that will produce amnesia. People vary on how the hypnotic experience affects them. In fact, some people have very clear memories of the trance process, while others simply enjoy the deep relaxation. But overall what you remember is up to you. If you are extremely focused then your memory will probably be crystal clear. And if you let your mind wander, then your memory of the experience will probably be hazy and dreamlike.

My favorite misconception is that only gullible or stupid people can be hypnotized. Quite the opposite! The smarter you are, the more likely you are to achieve a comfortable, relaxed and suggestive hypnotic state. The misconception probably became popular at the same time that Svengali was introduced. Think of Svengali as an all-powerful, goateed man waving a pocket watch slowly back and forth … back and forth … back and forth … (you are getting sleepy, are you not???), little by little leading his subject into a zombie-like state.

None of us want to be under the control of an all-powerful, mysterious character who by his will alone can command us to do his bidding. Anyone can be hypnotized if they wish to be, but it does require an ability to concentrate, focus, and follow directions. In case you weren't aware of it, all hypnosis is self-hypnosis. The hypnotist only acts like a tour guide and helps bring you into a hypnotic state through the use of carefully scripted words, phrases, and imagery. There is no coercion; there are no drugs and no tricks, and there is no magic.

Many theories have been put forward by both researchers and practitioners in the field of hypnotherapy as to the definition of hypnosis. Although hypnosis is generally defined as an altered state of consciousness (trance) that is enhanced through relaxation and the use of imagery, there is no commonly accepted definition of hypnosis. Here are just a few of the definitions put forth related to hypnosis:

"Hypnosis is largely a question of your willingness to be receptive and responsive to ideas, and to allow these ideas to act upon you without interference. These ideas we call suggestions." - Weitzenhoffer and Hilgard

"Hypnosis is a particular altered state of selective hyper-suggestibility brought about in an individual by the use of a combination of relaxation, fixation of attention and suggestion." - Ansari

"Hypnosis is a state of intensified attention and receptiveness to an idea or to a set of ideas." – Erickson

"Hypnosis is a state of relatively heightened susceptibility to prestige suggestions." - Clark Hull

"Hypnosis is a process which produces relaxation, distraction of the conscious mind, heightened suggestibility and increased awareness, allowing access to the subconscious mind through the imagination. It also produces the ability to experience thoughts and images as real." - A. M. Krasner

You can see by these quotations that over the years the experts have come up with many definitions. However, in all of these definitions hypnosis has the following similar ideas:

• There is an altered state

• Conscious / unconscious functioning occurs

• Suggestibility is heightened

A hypnotic state is a natural-occurring experience that is mixed in with our normal consciousness. Think of this naturally-occurring trance state as consisting of various levels that we can spontaneously enter and exit many times throughout the day. Daydreaming is probably the most well-known trance state and it shows up in many ways. Have you even been in a room full of people, but you were so lost in thought that you didn't understand what people said to you? Or sometimes you're just thinking of nothing and are completely unaware of the passage of time.

Driving trance is another form of daydreaming ... you know, you're driving home from somewhere and really don't remember how you got there or even what route you took because you were thinking about something else. There are other very common trance experiences, such as being absorbed in a book. When you're reading a book, the rest of the world disappears and you are a part of the world that the author has created for you. Let's take a quick look at some of the other natural-occurring states that are actually hypnotic experiences.

Age progression and age regression are two hypnotic experiences. During age progression (also called future-pacing) the hypnotist will have you vividly imagine yourself in the future. Maybe you want to be less anxious, or lose weight, or stop smoking, or reduce pain, or even reduce or eliminate your IBS symptoms.

You age progress yourself many times during a day. Maybe you're thinking about that party that is coming up this weekend, or maybe you're thinking about your summer wedding, or maybe you're thinking about living in that new house you just bought. All of these examples are a form of age progression.

Age regression is thinking about or reliving an event from the past. In Time Line Therapy, the practitioner will have a person go back into the past and pick up the learnings that they missed. This new learning removes, or at least changes, the emotion around painful memories. Any time you're thinking about something in the past, whether it's 2 minutes ago or 20 years ago, you are using age regression. You know … how about that lively discussion that happened at the meeting yesterday that you still think about. Or how about the pride that you feel each time you think about when you helped your friend last week when they really needed it. These are forms of age regression.

Amnesia is another hypnotic experience that occurs to you on a daily basis. You are subject to amnesia when you can't remember where you put your house keys, or when your next hypnotherapy appointment is, or what was the name of the person you were just introduced to at the party? Or have you ever been unsure whether you did something or just thought about needing to do it. You know, did you mail the house payment or were you just thinking about mailing it?

Confusion is one more naturally-occurring trance state. A confused person is in a trance of their own making because their conscious mind is preoccupied. Confusion is often intentionally utilized as a trance-inducing technique. During the time that the conscious mind is confused, it drops into what is called a transderivational search to make sense of what is being said or what has happened. While confused, the conscious mind is prone to draw upon unconscious learnings to make sense of things. Both Erickson and Rossi have stated that in their techniques, in fact almost all their techniques, there is confusion.

Dissociation is another naturally-occurring hypnotic phenomenon. Think of dissociation as "spacing out." When you're spaced out, your normal sensations and memories become altered. Very dissociated could be just losing your train of thought. In pain management, dissociation would be used to mentally separate the part of the body that is in pain from the rest of the body. Dissociation can also be used to distance a person from their unwanted emotions. Daydreaming is a form of dissociation. If you're remembering a favorite or an imagined place, then you are dissociating from the here and now and your five senses.

Negative and positive hallucinations are two other hypnotic experiences. Have you ever been at a friend's house for dinner and they asked you to look in the kitchen cabinet and get the salt shaker for them? You look and look and look and yell to them that it's not there. So what happens next? Your friend walks back into the room and grabs the salt shaker that's right there in front of your nose. That's a negative hallucination. It simply means that you do not perceive something that is actually there.

Have you ever had the experience of seeing someone out of the corner of your eye, but when you look directly for them they seem to have vanished? That's a positive hallucination. Positive hallucinations are the opposite of negative hallucinations, that is, positive hallucinations are when you perceive something that is not actually there. When you're daydreaming about someone or some situation, then you are creating a positive hallucination. You might notice that positive hallucinations are very similar to age progression.

Post-Hypnotic Suggestions are a main part of hypnosis and something that you do all the time. In hypnotic terms, a post-hypnotic suggestion is a "command" given while a person is under hypnosis that will be acted upon later in their full waking state. Every form of hypnotherapy uses hypnotic suggestions. In everyday terms, a post-hypnotic suggestion is usually something you remind yourself to do later. How many times do you say something like, "I need to pick up something for dinner before I go home." Or, "I need to get gas before I go to visit my parents."

Sensory modification is yet another hypnotic experience. This is one of the important techniques for pain management. Sensory modification is something that you do naturally. Think of a time when a person came into your office or your home and they had on too much perfume or cologne. At first the smell was overwhelming, but over time you hardly noticed it. This is a decreasing of your sensory awareness. Some people live close to a railroad, and over time the passing of trains fades off into the distance. Or maybe you're in earshot of the county fair, and when you first notice it, it's very loud. Other people may comment on it; however within a short period of time it's totally out of your conscious awareness.

So you can see that probably 100% of the population (including yourself) experiences trance in some form or another on a daily basis.

You may think that hypnosis has not been around for very long. Maybe you think it's some type of new-age technique. Well it turns out that hypnosis, or what's also known as the trance state, has been with us since the dawn of time. In the next chapter we'll hit some of the highlights of hypnosis related to healing, imagination, and expectancy.

19

A BRIEF HISTORY OF
HYPNOSIS AND HYPNOTISM

Hypnosis has been practiced for thousands of years, and is one of the oldest forms of medicine and healing by trance state (hypnosis). Hypnosis has been practiced under an assortment of diverse pretexts to heal the sick since ancient times. The earliest medical records describe inexplicable healing brought about in a sleep-like state by priests or demigods in the Aesculapian temples of ancient Greece. Asclepius was the Greco-Roman god of medicine. It was said that Asclepius could cure the sick in dreams, so the practice of sleeping in his temples became common. It may be of some interest that Asclepius is often represented holding a staff with a serpent coiled around it, which is the dominant symbol for professional healthcare associations in the United States.

Ancient Sanskrit writings also describe the use of trance and healing temples in India. The ancient Egyptians and Greeks used sleep temples, where sleep and incantations were used, and these sleep temples are also well-documented. Sleep temples were even used hundreds of years later during the Roman Empire. Hippocrates and Hippocratic medicine are descendants of this form of medicine.

Let's move up to the 1500s where a Swiss medical doctor named Paracelsus (who discovered the mercury cure for syphilis), was also using visualization for healing. Paracelsus said, "As man imagines himself to be, so shall he be, and he is that which he imagines." He was also the first physician known to use magnets (or lodestones) for healing.

The beginning of modern hypnosis is associated with two men: Mesmer from whom the term *mesmerism* came, and the Scottish surgeon James Braid whom we will discuss later.

Mesmer, Imagination, and the Law of Expectancy

I want to go into a little more depth in covering Mesmer because his work bridges the gap between, imagination, expectation, and hypnosis, all of which you will need to understand to make significant changes to your IBS symptoms.

In Mesmer's day, physicians used techniques such as of blistering, enemas, and purgatives. Bloodletting was also one of the major interventions. After opening a patient's vein, Mesmer would make passes over the cut with a magnet, and the bleeding would stop. Unfortunately (or fortunately) one time when Mesmer was bleeding a patient, he reached for his magnets and could not find them. So instead of using a magnetic, he grabbed a stick and used it to pass over the patient's cut ... and interestingly enough the bleeding still stopped! Today in terms of hypnosis, we would suggest (no pun intended, well maybe just a little) that passing the magnet or stick was simply imparting a non-verbal suggestion causing trance to occur which has therapeutic benefits. Mesmer called this energy *Animal Magnetism,* and that name would eventually discredit Mesmer.

Mesmer's results were often quite remarkable, curing people of nearly every problem, and many patients would have hysterical reactions. Patients would cry out or begin to convulse by wildly flailing their limbs. Many of them went into a state of drowsiness, or sleep. And once they had "awakened," his patients would report feeling much better and appeared to have been cured. Soon everyone who was anyone went to Dr. Mesmer for one of his magnetic cures, including those in the royal court. One person in the royal court that you might be familiar with was Marie Antoinette.

In Paris around 1784, Mesmer's reputation grew so large that his unorthodox methods and the tremendous fame of his dramatic cures not only earned the strong anger and denouncements by the French medical community, but King Louis XVI also became worried that Mesmer was becoming more important that he was! Most "respected" physicians disregarded the success that Mesmer was having with his patients because the physicians felt that Mesmer's noninvasive dramatic techniques were nothing more than hocus-pocus.

The French medical community wanted to discredit Mesmer, so besides not accepting him or his techniques, they warned King Louis XVI of a danger. This danger was a mysterious force that no one had actually seen, but it had vast power. It turns out that the name of this danger had two names: expectation, and imagination.

In the name of science, King Louis XVI appointed a royal commission to investigate mesmerism, and this invisible animal magnetism stuff. The commission contained four people who are famous today: Antoine Lavoisier (the father of modern chemistry); Jean-Sylvain Bailly (the astronomer, who calculated the orbit of Halley's Comet); the famous American Benjamin Franklin; and a medical doctor who was an expert in pain control named Joseph-Ignace Guillotin yes, that Guillotin).

The commission was not interested in the effects of this animal magnetic healing; instead they were interested in determining if magnetism was responsible for Mesmer's cures. **They did not care to investigate if the patients were in fact being healed**. What they were interested in was whether or not Mesmer was a fraud and magnetic healing treatments were dishonest.

The commission failed to discover any tangible and material evidence, so the practice of animal magnetism became illegal. Franklin wrote the majority opinion to the King which said, "The experience is therefore entirely conclusive ... this fellow Mesmer is not flowing anything from his hands that I can see. Therefore, this mesmerism must be a fraud." Magnetic **healing was caused by imagination and expectations,** not by some mysterious universal energy.

D'Eslon was Mesmer's protégé, and a preeminent doctor and precursor of the modern 19th Century thinker that believed in alternative healing. D'Eslon believed in the concept of a universal healing energy and had written a letter to his fellow doctors defending Mesmer. D'Elson stated:

> " ... *if Monsieur Mesmer had no other secret than to be able to cause the imagination to act effectively to produce health, would he not have a marvelous thing?*"

Interestingly enough, the answer from the French physicians about using imagination as a way to produce health was met with a resounding NO that still resonates today. Not only did the physicians believe, but the members of the commission also believed, that imagination was an "active and terrible power." The report described imagination as a cross between charlatan and bogeyman, and to call upon it was to dabble in the dark arts.

OK, let's continue your journey trying to stay away from the shadows and superstitions as we move ahead with our investigation of the story of hypnosis and hypnotherapy. Let's look at James Braid.

James Braid (1795-1860), coined the term "hypnosis" from the Greek Hypnos (meaning sleep). He first became interested in mesmerism in 1840 when he went to see a demonstration by a mesmerist named

La Fontaine. Braid did not believe that mesmerism (trance) had anything to do with magnetic fluids or the transfer of energy. The mesmerist La Fontaine would stand near the head of the patient and make downward hand passes over the body. What intrigued Braid was that the patient's eyes would remain locked while staring at La Fontaine. Braid realized the importance of the eyes being fixated in causing trance and introduced the technique of visual fixation and eye fatigue to induce hypnosis.

Braid also deduced that mesmerism worked because of the combination of eye fixation and suggestion and these two together caused the patient to go into trance. Trance then, was a state brought on by tiring the eyes, causing a condition that resembles sleep. In 1843, Braid published the first book on hypnosis entitled, *Neurypnology*, (also known as the Rationale of Nervous Sleep Considered in Relation to Animal Magnetism). In that book he spelled out that the fixation on a single point or idea is what causes hypnosis to occur.

Braid later understood that hypnosis was not the right term because the trance state had nothing to do with sleep. He later tried to change the name to *Monoideaism*, which did not do any better than *Neurypnology*. Braid may have gotten the original name wrong, but he did intuitively sense what we practitioners in the field of hypnosis know today, and that is that the trance state is a combination of the effects of the hypnotist's suggestions along with the unconscious responses of the client.

You may not know this but Freud also originally was interested and used hypnosis. The young Sigmund Freud (1856-1939) studied at the Nancy School where he observed posthypnotic suggestions being carried out by the patients after they had been hypnotized. He also gained insight into hidden memories and their effect on human behavior. Freud initially used hypnosis in his practice to uncover these hidden memories, but later found that he had more success in getting patients to talk about these forgotten memories without actually hypnotizing them. It is said that the reason that Freud stopped using hypnosis was that a young female patient had jumped up and kissed him. However, it could be that Freud stopped using hypnosis because his use of cocaine damaged his gums, causing his false teeth to not fit well, which affected his ability to speak well enough to induce trance easily. Freud may also have quit using hypnosis because he was in competition with a Viennese Physician named Dr. Josef Breuer (1842-1925) who was an excellent hypnotist.

Freud created the "talking therapy," which he said would not be a therapy for the poor, and it would take 100 to 300 hours to effect a cure. At one 1-hour session per week, this talking cure would take between two to six years to take effect. This talking therapy that Freud described became psychoanalysis. Freudian psychoanalysis became so popular in psychology that it actually became inappropriate to use any other technique. Consequently, hypnosis went "out of vogue."

Emile Coue (1857-1926), a European pharmacologist, developed an idea known today as autosuggestion. Coue found that patients responded more positively to prescribed medication if he put emphasis on the medicine's effectiveness. From this observation, he suggested that unconscious responses can be affected by using imagination. The popularity of self-hypnosis can be traced back and credited to Coue.

In 1955, hypnosis for anesthesia received a revival from the British Medical Association (BMA). The BMA declared that,

"There is a place for hypnotism in the production of anesthesia or analgesia for surgery and dental operations, and in suitable subjects it is an effective method of relieving

pains in childbirth without altering the normal course of labor."

In 1958, the American Medical Association (AMA) sanctioned the use of hypnotism by physicians while remaining critical of using hypnosis for entertainment purposes.

For the first part of the 20th century, there were not any impressive advancements in hypnosis. Everything seemed rather dull, until in 1933 when Clark Leonard Hull (1884-1952), while employed as a research professor of psychology at Yale University, published his classic work *Hypnosis and Suggestibility.* Hull was not a hypnotherapist by any definition of the word; he was an academic and scientist. This landmark text helped shape the progression and advancement of hypnosis. Hull believed that,

"Anything that assumes trance, causes trance,"

and it is this fundamental principle that makes anything possible in creating hypnosis. From this point of view, Neuro-linguistic Programming (NLP), guided imagery, and even visualization are hypnosis. Hull is also significant because of his inspiration and encouragement on the young Milton Erickson, who was present at some of Hull's early researches.

Milton H. Erickson MD. (1901-1980), is almost certainly the most famous American hypnotherapist of the second half of the 20th century. He practiced hypnosis on a regular basis from 1920 until his death in 1980. Erickson's techniques, especially his acute observation skills, his use of artfully vague language, and his story telling ability, had a major impact on using hypnosis in therapy. Using these techniques would cause a patient's problem to disappear as if by magic. Erickson's approach became a major part of the original work known as Neuro-linguistic Programming (NLP).

Today, hypnosis has expanded its horizons and moved into new territories, particularly due to advances in brain imaging technology. Thanks to the help of brain imaging technology, hypnotic suggestions have been shown to have an effect on perception. A simple example of this comes from a study conducted at Stanford University (*"Hypnotic Visual Illusion Alters Color Processing In The Brain"*). Subjects were given the suggestion that the black-and-white photo they were looking at was actually in color. And can you guess what happened according to the brain scans? The brain scans showed that the color processing areas of the brain were activated, even though the subjects were viewing a black-and-white photo! This demonstrates that the mind cannot tell the difference between something that is vividly imagined compared to something that is "real."

OK, now that you have some background and understand the importance of expectation and imagery, let's find out what it's like to have a hypnotherapy session.

20

WHAT SHOULD YOU EXPECT DURING YOUR HYPNOTHERAPY SESSION?

You have moved past superstition and fears related to hypnosis and now you're curious to find out if hypnosis and hypnotherapy can really help you reduce or even eliminate your IBS symptoms. At some point you will be interested in using hypnotherapy, so let's go over what you should expect during your first hypnotherapy appointment related to IBS.

Besides taking a detailed personal history, the hypnotherapist will usually quickly go over the misconceptions about hypnosis, which you are now completely familiar with. One of the goals of the first session is to make sure that you feel at ease, and that you have a conscious willingness to change. Problems will be explored, beliefs and habits will be identified, and expected outcomes will be set. Finding out what your expectations are related to your IBS symptoms are extremely important. Hypnotherapy is a co-operative working arrangement between the client (which is you) and the hypnotherapist; think of it as working together in a therapeutic partnership.

Hypnotherapy has a "structure". It relies on a formal or informal induction, which can be achieved by an assortment of methods. Sometimes just the speed and tone of the hypnotherapist's voice is enough to lead you into deep relaxation. Once you achieve a relaxed state (and probably a sense of dissociation), possibly though the use of imagery or suggestions, the trance state can be "deepened" by a number of techniques; however, a medium depth of trance is all that is required for good therapeutic results. This is followed by therapeutic interventions using a mixture of analogies, direct or indirect suggestions, and metaphors related to changing some aspect of the your mental or physical functioning.

At this point there might be a review or compounding of the suggestions used. Post hypnotic suggestions can be used, as well as "future pacing." Future pacing is also called mental rehearsal and it's the process of going out into the future (which could be a day, a week, six months, six years, etc.) to a time when you have successfully made the changes that you wish. You would see yourself in a situation performing and acting according to your new "programming." In the case of IBS, you would see yourself free from living your life around IBS symptoms, and living a "normal" life.

The last "step" in the session is to emerge you from the trance state. Sometimes this is called "awaken", but basically the hypnotist will reorient you back to your normal state of awareness. Some schools of hypnosis do not like to use either the word sleep or awaken because they feel that this propagates the notion that hypnosis is related to sleep. Emerging can be done by counting you back up and making suggestions that you will be completely alert.

OK, that's typically what happens in a hypnotic session, but how does hypnosis work? First off, scientists cannot agree on precisely how hypnosis works. The theory is that in the hypnotic state, the conscious mind is off doing something and its power of judgment is either fully or partially suppressed. There seems to be a slight transfer away from the critical, judging, analytical, conscious processes involving the left cerebral hemisphere function towards the creative and imaginative unconscious processes, involving the right hemisphere. This is what is meant when you hear that, "Hypnosis is an altered state of consciousness." Your attention is being "altered" from the judgmental left-hand side of the brain to the non-judgmental right-hand side of the brain. This shift allows suggestions to by-pass the conscious mind's "critical faculty" allowing suggestions to freely enter into the unconscious mind with little or no interruption from the conscious mind. This hyper-suggestibility appears to be an important factor.

Think of the critical faculty like the gatekeeper that stands between the conscious mind and the unconscious mind. The gatekeeper's responsibility is to only allow information through that is consistent with the unconscious mind's programming. Before the gatekeeper is given a job to do, there is not much information in the unconscious mind to be inconsistent with, so most information becomes new programming. The gatekeeper develops around the age of four, five, or six and it decides what information gets through and will become a program that runs in the unconscious mind. Once programming has been established, then the gatekeeper will disregard any suggestion that is contrary to the information that is already stored. If the suggestion is in line with the unconscious programming then the suggestion is allowed complete access to the unconscious mind. So to change old programming, the gatekeeper (critical faculty) needs to be bypassed and that's what hypnosis does.

But why do we need "direct" access to the unconscious mind? Well, your automatic responses (breathing, or gut transit speed for example), habits, and long-term memories are stored in your unconscious mind. Hypnosis works with your unconscious mind because that is where those old habits, memories, and "programs" are stored. Hypnosis goes directly to the source to make the changes that the client wants and feels are appropriate.

Of course it is assumed that the person wants the suggestions that are being given. The suggestions need to be in the best interest of the client so that they are able to accept and integrate new behaviors, beliefs, concepts, ideas and thoughts.

Suggestions for change can be given by using metaphors, or imagery, or by using hypnotic language patterns, or even by using direct authoritative suggestions. It is said that we are unable to distinguish between something "real" or something vividly imagined. And the suggestions are meant to persuade the unconscious mind that the suggestions are true and will occur.

While in this altered state, the patient's attention is focused on, and has a heightened sensitivity to, one particular thing (or closely-related things), and at the same time, a decreased awareness of other activities or sounds going on around them. The success of hypnotic suggestions varies based on the client's belief, and on the words and phrases being used.

By the very "structure" of a hypnotic session, you can see that many beneficial elements are being used. Various studies indicate that the activity of breathing tends to affect the many parts of the autonomic nervous system. During relaxation breathing is slow, deep, and has a regular rhythm, which activates parasympathetic processes. Relaxation has an important role in reducing stress. I always suggest to my clients that they can expect to feel the most relaxed that they have ever felt while being in the (trance) chair, and no they can't take the chair home with them! Because the autonomic nervous system is predisposed to imitating what's happening with your breathing, relaxed breathing then becomes a way to gain control over "automatic" physiological processes.

Hypnosis also sets the expectation that their psychological problems or old (bad) habits will be resolved. Of particular relevance to you as an IBS sufferer, is that the hypnotic state allows you to influence your physiological mechanisms, such as gut transit speed, gut pain sensitivity, immune responsiveness, and the level of activity of your GI tract.

You know enough about hypnosis now to realize that the mind is able to affect the body. So since that is true, the question that you're probably asking yourself is, "**Can it help me** with my IBS symptoms?" Well, read on and you'll become convinced that the answer to your question is a resounding **YES!**

21

CAN MIND-BODY COMMUNICATION AFFECT IBS SYMPTOMS?

Psychological therapies, including hypnotherapy, are hardly ever recommended to IBS patients. Health professionals typically focus on the cause of disease rather than on what promotes health. Besides changes in diet, the standard medical methods currently used to treat Irritable Bowel Syndrome, such as antidiarrheals, antidepressants, antispasmodics, and laxatives have been the treatment of choice. This type of treatment helps only a small minority of IBS patients. It's no wonder that more than half[1] of IBS sufferers are dissatisfied with the results of standard medical management. It seems that psychological interventions are a logical choice because the brain helps regulate GI function and also controls pain perception in the gut.

Interest in the mind-body connection continues growing because past and current research has shown a vast amount of evidence demonstrating that connections exist between the brain, immune system, and nervous system. Communication between these different areas are bi-directionally and use cytokines (small molecules used for cell signaling), hormones, and neuropeptides. Previously, the brain, immune system, and nervous system, had been thought of as being independent, but there is an overwhelming amount of credible data that the effects of hypnosis (through expectation, imagery, and visualization) are able to influence both the immune system and nervous system.

So how can hypnotherapy help IBS sufferers? Let's first look at what we know is possible with hypnotherapy.

Hypnotherapy is a complementary treatment which has been proved effective over a wide range of disorders, both physical and psychological, such as allergies, the alleviation of pain, anxiety, cancer, childbirth (hypnosis, on average, reduces childbirth time by four hours), depression, functional dyspepsia (indigestion), GI disorders, and phobias to name just a few.

GI disorders that include pain, nausea, and vomiting show up a lot in the medical profession. Chemotherapy can cause it, various medications can cause it, and pregnancy can cause nausea and vomiting. Numerous studies have shown that hypnosis reduces or alleviates pain, nausea and vomiting.

Hypnosis and pain relief are one of the most researched areas (Lynn et al.[2]). Hypnosis has the ability to adjust and modify the psychological experience of pain. Hypnoanalgesia is one of the more powerful techniques used in hypnosis for the management of pain. For most people, hypnoanalgesia will decrease both acute and chronic pain.

For acute pain, hypnosis has proven effective in surgical procedures such as appendectomies, bone marrow aspiration, the treatment of burns (dressing changes and the painful removal of dead or contaminated skin tissue), child-birth labor pain, dental work, interventional radiology (minimally-invasive procedures to diagnose and treat diseases in nearly every organ system), and tumor excisions. For patients who receive hypnotherapy before surgical procedures, they can expect reduced anxiety, less blood loss, reduced pain, and a lower incidence of post-operative nausea and vomiting.

For chronic pain, hypnosis has been proven effective for conditions such as backache, fibromyalgia, headache, and TMJ.

So let's look at some data related to hypnosis and pain.

In 2003, a review of controlled clinical studies using hypnoanalgesia was evaluated by Patterson and Jensen[3]. The review found that hypnoanalgesia is valuable for significant reductions in things like the length of time a patient stays in a hospital, or the patient's ratings of pain. Hypnoanalgesia also reduces that patient's need for analgesics or sedation, as well as reducing nausea and vomiting. Patients treated with hypnosis consistently rate higher levels of satisfaction with their care compared to patients who only received standard care. Patterson and Jensen went further with their conclusions by saying that hypnotic techniques are equal or more effective than other treatments for both acute and chronic pain. Not only does hypnosis save both money and time for patients and clinicians, but evidence indicates that hypnosis might be considered a standard of treatment, unless of course, the person shows a strong resistance to it.

In 1999, neuropsychologist Rainville et al.,[4] reported that according to their brain imaging research, patients with moderate suggestibility (which makes up the majority of people) and of course highly receptive patients, found long-lasting relief from hypnosis techniques.

In 2000, a meta-analysis of 18 published pain studies was evaluated by Montgomery et al.[5] The analysis confirmed that hypnotic techniques provided a substantial amount of pain relief in 75% of clinical and experimental participants. The analysis also confirmed that hypnosis would likely be effective no matter what type of pain the patient was experiencing.

Studies in the field of cancer demonstrated the effect that hypnosis has on the immune system. In 1978 the first research into end-stage cancer treatments and hypnosis was carried out (see Simonton, 1978, *Getting Well Again*).

I brought up indigestion (functional dyspepsia) a moment ago, so let's look at another study. A study in 2002 by Calvert et al.,[6] investigated hypnotherapy for the treatment of indigestion. Originally 126 patients were randomly assigned into three groups: hypnotherapy, supportive therapy plus placebo medication, or medical treatment. 26 hypnotherapy patients, 24 supportive therapy plus placebo medication patients, and 29 medical treatment patients completed all phases of the study. Results were taken at 16 weeks, and again at 56 weeks. Quality of life (QOL) was also measured as a secondary result.

The results pointed out that the hypnotherapy group improved more in both the short-term (16 week) and long-term (56 week) compared to the other two groups. Long-term results showed the largest variance between the hypnotherapy group and the other groups. After 56 weeks the hypnotherapy group had significantly improved symptoms (73%) compared with medical treatment (43%), or supportive therapy plus placebo medication (34%).

The hypnotherapy group had a QOL improvement of 44% compared to the medical treatment groups 20%. The supportive therapy plus placebo medication group did have a 43% improvement; however, five of the patients were taking antidepressants. No patient in the hypnotherapy group started taking medication during follow-up compared to 82% of the patients in the supportive therapy group and 90% in the medical treatment group. Taking into account repeated visits to medical doctors, and the high cost of medication, patients would get a huge benefit from hypnotherapy.

What about hypnosis and emotions? Can hypnosis change the intensity of your emotions, and if it can will that reduce your IBS symptoms?

The undesirable effect of emotions on physical health, and the connection between mind and body and the influence that one has on the other is not a new idea. Hippocrates trained his students to think about their patient's life circumstances and emotions. In the second century, the Greek physician Galen observed that discontented or sad women were more inclined to be affected by malignancies of the breast than cheerful women.

The brain translates attitudes, beliefs, feelings, memories, thoughts, and values into multifaceted patterns of chemical release and nerve cell firing that affect the biochemistry and physiology of the body. Emotions such as anger, anxiety, fear, and pain, have shown to affect colonic motility and rectal sensitivity, more so in IBS sufferers than in healthy controls. Hypnosis reduces colonic motility and normalizes rectal sensitivity, which would be expected to improve GI function.

Mental states affect the function of the GI tract in both people with and without IBS symptoms. Since negative states have a negative impact on the GI tract, it seems that positive states should have a positive calming effect.

To further set your expectations, it's time to look at a few studies that were done, related to mind-body approaches and hypnosis.

22

SUMMARIZING THE MIND-BODY APPROACH

If you're like most people with IBS, you have spent enough time researching information, whether it's about diet, or medications, or current strategies for treating IBS. You're just looking for the right information, that magic bullet that will bring back your quality of life. Most people however, want some solid proof about hypnotherapy and the mind-body approach, so let's take a look at some of the published reports.

Hypnotherapy utilizes a number of mind-body therapies and the literature supporting mind-body therapies is highly persuasive. Hypnotherapy for the treatment of IBS uses various forms of relaxation (such as progressive relaxation, and meditation), imagery, positive suggestion, therapeutic suggestions on recording (the original ones were on audiotape), and therapy.

In 1987, Voirol and Hipolito et al.,[1] found that relaxation not only reduced symptoms but also prevented relapse. In 1993 Blanchard, Greene, and Scharff[2], and in 2001 and 2002, Keefer and Blanchard[3, 4] reported similar findings.

In 1992, Guthrie and Creed et al.,[5] created a study with patients who had not responded to medication alone. Their approach was to add relaxation and therapy to the patients that were already taking medication. They found that two-thirds of the patients had symptom reductions. Keefer and Blanchard in 2002 also reported that relaxation (in the form of meditation) was able to affect improvements that were maintained a year later.

Confirming the power of the mind-body connection, in 2004, Simren and Ringstrom et al.,[6] conducted a study with 28 patients showing the superiority of hypnotherapy compared to a supportive therapy control group in reducing the sensory and motor component of the gastrocolonic response in IBS. The hypnotherapy group consisted of nine females and five males that ranged in age from 25 to 67 years. In this group three had diarrhea-predominant IBS (IBS-D), two had constipation-predominant IBS (IBS-C), and nine had alternating diarrhea and constipation (IBS-M), according to Rome II criteria. The hypnotherapy group had twice as many patients reporting improvements (71.4%) compared to the control group (35.7%).

Many case studies have shown that hypnosis improves symptoms even in severe refractory cases. A few of these studies are listed here: Francis and Houghton, 1996[7]; Galovski and Blanchard, 1998[8]; Forbes, MacAulay, and Chiotakakou-Faliakou, 2000[9]; Houghton et al., 2002[10]; Barabasz A, Barabasz M, 2006[11]; Roberts and Wilson et al., 2006[12].

Other studies have shown that hypnotherapy was successful with IBS patients where psychotherapy had failed (Whorwell, Prior, and Faragher, 1984[13]).

In 1998, Galovsky et al.,[14] and in 2000 Forbes et al.,[15] finished studies in gut-directed hypnotherapy suggestion. They concluded that hypnotherapy created significant symptom improvement. The Forbes study investigated the effect of therapeutic suggestions on audiotape and found the recordings effective; in fact, the audio recordings were more than twice as effective as making changing to the patient's diet and adding medications.

In 1983, Svedlund and Sjodin et al.,[16] showed that IBS patients receiving medication deteriorated, while IBS patients receiving therapy improved. In 2002, Svendlun[17] reviewed 22 studies and found that in 19 of the studies, therapy was superior to medication.

In 1987, Blanchard and Radnitz et al.,[18] demonstrated the effectiveness of mind-body techniques in not only reducing IBS's physical symptoms, but also in lifting depression and improving quality of life. This was also reported by Houghton, Heyman, and Whorwell in 1996[19], Read in 1999[20], and Gonsasalkorale, Toner, and Whorwell in 2004[21].

The value of hypnotherapy for not only IBS but for the comorbity factors was also established in 2002 by Gonsalkorale, Houghton, and Whorwell[22]. A large-scale British study of 250 patients confirmed that hypnosis significantly improved not only IBS symptoms, but anxiety, depression, and quality of life also improved.

In 1991, a strong mind-body part to IBS was demonstrated by Whorwell and Houghton et al.[23] They (along with Salt and Neimark[24] later in 2002) also demonstrated that emotions have an effect on gut motility. Also in 2002, Houghton and Calvert et al.,[25] showed that hypnotically induced anger and excitement increased the motility of the colon, whereas happiness reduced motility.

OK, now I want you to get deep into the bowels (no pun intended, well maybe just a little) of a number of studies that were done using hypnosis in the treatment of IBS. Let's jump into our "way-back" machine and look at the studies that go back to 1984. Also, research today continues to investigate hypnosis in the treatment of IBS. You're about to see (and your expectation will continue to strengthen) that based on these studies you can use the power of gut-directed hypnotherapy to change your IBS symptoms!

23

WHY USE
GUT-DIRECTED HYPNOSIS
FOR THE TREATMENT OF IBS?

You know that dietary modification and prescribed medications are effective for only about 25% of IBS sufferers. To put it another way, that means that 75% of IBS sufferers do not respond to traditional treatment. That sure sounds like it's worth investigating a different method of treatment.

So what if there was a treatment that had a clinically reported success rate of 70% to 90%? Would that be of value to you, as a person that has been diagnosed with IBS? Well, there are many, many (did I say many?) clinical studies that confirm that using hypnotherapy for the treatment of IBS can do exactly that!

Think about this for a moment: besides promoting relaxation, hypnosis can be used to alleviate pain. Hypnosis has also been shown to affect smooth muscle activity, so it only makes sense that hypnosis would have a successful role in the treatment of IBS. Hypnosis is also effective in reducing stress, and although it has not been found that IBS symptoms are caused directly by stress, research tells us that psychological stress intensifies IBS symptoms.

Psychological stress is caused by how the mind interprets what is happening around it. For people with IBS, negative interpretation leads to problems with how the GI tract is functioning. It seems like if the mind had a positive interpretation, then it would have a calming and peaceful influence on the GI tract.

In case you didn't know this, gut-directed hypnotherapy is the most frequently reported therapy shown to have a favorable beneficial influence on IBS symptoms. But where did it all begin? The "way-back" machine should be warmed up by now, so let's go back in time to 1984 and see where this all started. Let's look at the gut-directed hypnotherapy treatment that was first described by the Manchester group in 1984 (Whorwell PJ, et al.[1]).

In a randomized controlled trial, 26 women and 4 men between 25 to 53 years of age, whom had all been under Whorwell's care for at least one year, were given either gut-directed hypnotherapy, or psychotherapy plus placebo.

For the purposes of this study, IBS was defined by the existence of abdominal distension, abdominal pain, and an uncharacteristic bowel habit, such as constipation, diarrhea, or alternating diarrhea and constipation. Also, all biochemistry and hematology had to be normal, and contrast radiography or colonoscopy had to be normal also.

Sometimes a sizeable placebo response is a trait of clinical trials in IBS, and this might be anticipated to occur in an "unconventional" form of treatment such as hypnotherapy. To minimize any placebo response, all patients selected for this study had already proved refractory, that is, they had not responded to bulking and spasmolytic agents and had not responded in at least one previous controlled therapeutic trial. On average, each of the 30 patients had received six different types of therapies per patient and none had responded to any type of treatment.

Dr. Whorwell conducted interventions for both groups, each of which consisted of seven half-hour sessions of decreasing frequency over a three-month period. After the third session, patients were given an audio tape that contained suggestions similar to those given in the session for daily autohypnosis. Hypnotherapy was exclusively directed at general relaxation and control of intestinal motility, and no effort was made at hypnoanalysis. Hypnoanalysis is the use of hypnosis in conjunction with psychoanalytic techniques.

Before hypnosis, the patient was given a simple education of intestinal-smooth-muscle physiology (for more information see the chapter called, "Introduction To Your Digestive System"). Hypnosis was induced by an arm-levitation technique followed by various deepening techniques based upon the patient's progress and visualization abilities. After general suggestions for improvement of health and well-being, focus was aimed at controlling the patient's intestinal smooth muscle. Suggestions were then given. One of the suggestions used for controlling gut function was to have the patient place their hand on their abdomen and be aware of a feeling of warmth as they pictured and imagined their gut as a smoothly flowing river. All hypnotherapy sessions concluded with standard ego-strengthening suggestions, as well as suggestions for the health and well-being of the patient.

One group received seven half-hour supportive psychotherapy sessions from Whorwell plus a placebo. The supportive psychotherapy sessions incorporated conversations about the patient's symptoms and an investigation about any possible contributory emotional problems and stressful life events.

All patients were required to keep a daily diary card on which they recorded the frequency and severity of abdominal distension and pain. Bowel habits were also recorded and abnormality was expressed. These rating were as follows:

3 = severe

2 = moderate

1 = mild

0 = none

Symptom improvement and well-being were scored each week on a 3 to 0 scale, with 3 indicating maximum improvement and 0 indicating no improvement.

By the end of the study, IBS symptoms (abdominal distension, abdominal pain, bowel habits, and well-being) were either mild or absent in all 15 hypnotherapy patients. The overall improvements were significantly greater in the hypnotherapy group than in the psychotherapy plus placebo group.

Except for bowel habits, the psychotherapy plus placebo group reported a small but significant improvement in all symptoms. The disparity between the two groups reached significance by the fourth week of treatment for abdominal distension, bowel habit, and well-being, and significance for abdominal pain was reached by the fifth week of treatment.

This study was probably the first to demonstrate that hypnotherapy is highly effective in the treatment of refractory IBS. And as a note, no replacement symptoms were observed during or after the study. What was unusual about this study is that an improvement in all symptoms was found. Typically, not ALL symptoms in a study will be improved. Whorwell et al.,[2] did a follow-up study to evaluate the long-term effects of these patients.

Here are a couple of charts adapted from Whorwell et al., *Lancet*, 1984 2:1232-4 showing how well hypnosis as a treatment for IBS performed, compared to the psychotherapy plus placebo group.

Abdominal Pain

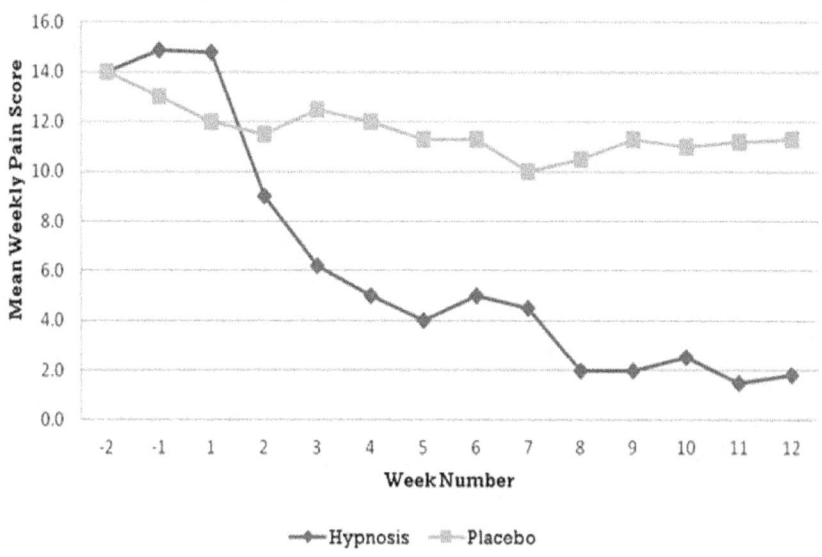

As you can see from the abdominal pain chart, the psychotherapy plus placebo group started at the beginning of the study (shown as -1) with a pain score of about 13, and the hypnotherapy group started with a pain score of about 15. At the end of 12 weeks, the psychotherapy plus placebo group showed a slight change down to 12 in their pain score, and the hypnotherapy group significantly decreased their pain score to about 2, which is around an 86% reduction!

Abdominal Distention

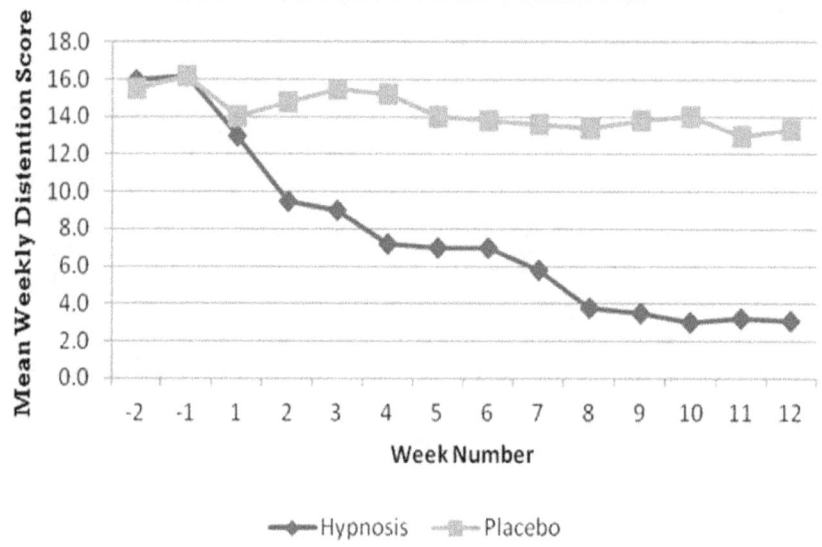

The abdominal distention chart at the beginning of the study (shown as -1) shows that the psychotherapy plus placebo group started at a distention score of about 16, and the hypnotherapy group started with about the same pain score. At the end of 12 weeks, the psychotherapy plus placebo group had a slight change in their distention score (to about 13.5), and the hypnotherapy group decreased their distention score to about 3, which is about an 81% reduction!

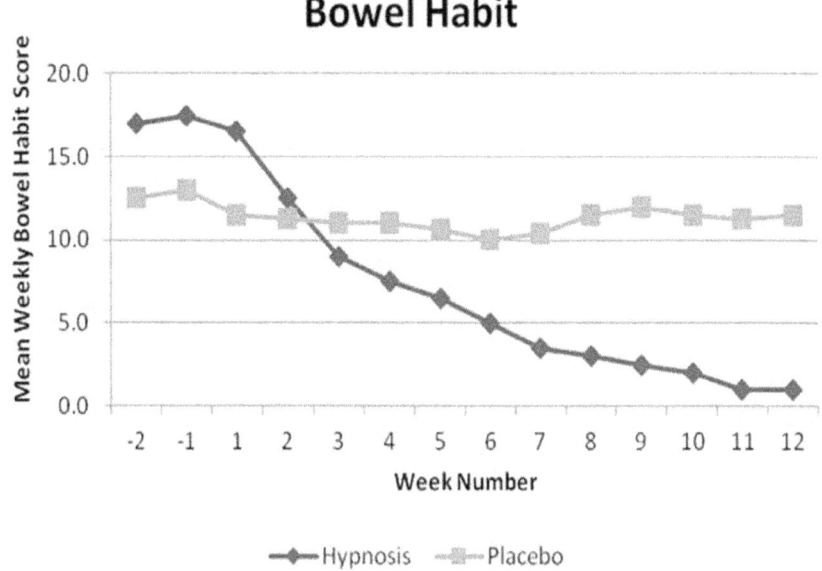

Bowel Habit

The bowel habit chart at the beginning of the study (shown as -1) shows that the psychotherapy plus placebo group started with a bowel habit score of about 12.5, and the hypnotherapy group started with a bowel score of about 17.5. At the end of 12 weeks, the psychotherapy plus placebo group had a slight change in their bowel habit score, and the hypnotherapy group decreased their bowel habit score to about 1, which is about a 97% reduction!

Well Being

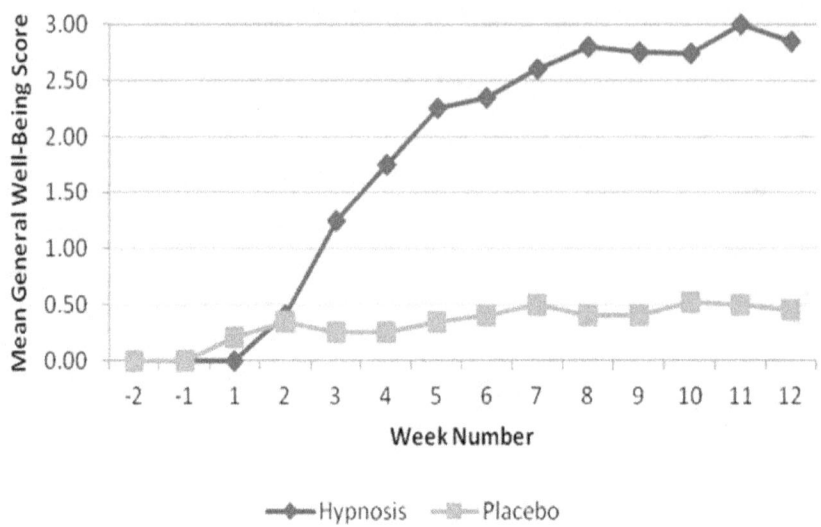

Hypnosis ——— Placebo

The well-being chart shows that the psychotherapy plus placebo group started at the beginning of the study (week -1) with a well-being score of about 0, and the hypnotherapy group started with the same score. At the end of 12 weeks, the psychotherapy plus placebo scores showed a very slight improvement with their well-being score moving up to about 0.5. The hypnotherapy group increased their well-being score to about 2.8. Remember the top of the well-being score was set at 3.

The original 15 hypnotherapy patients were followed for an average of 18 months and had "tune-up" sessions every third month. During the 18-month follow-up period two patients had a return of symptoms. These patients were successfully treated with an extra session of hypnotherapy. At the conclusion of the follow-up period, all patients remained in remission with symptoms not meaningfully different from the results of the original study.

During this same study, 35 new patients (31 women, 4 men, aged 23 to 65) with severe IBS symptoms who had proved refractory to conventional forms of treatment were added to the study and divided into one of three groups. All patients received hypnotherapy.

The study now had 50 patients. One group of seven patients was called the atypical group because they were lacking one or two of the three symptoms mandatory to be classified as a classical case. Another group of 38 patients was called classical cases because they had abdominal distension, abdominal pain, and disturbed bowel habits. And the third group of five patients was made up of patients with classical IBS plus significant coexisting psychopathology. The original study only included patients that would have fallen into the classical cases group.

The results of these now 50 patients were evaluated as "improved" only if their symptoms were rated as a 1 = mild, or 0 = none, and they required no medication for IBS, except bulking agents were allowed. Two of "non-responders" (which happened to be women) failed to complete their daily diary card and were assumed to have severe symptoms for the purposes of the study.

The overall success rate was 84% (remember this means that they reported either mild of no symptoms), with patients reporting significant improvements in abdominal distension, abdominal pain, bowel habits, and general well-being. In the atypical patients group, 43% responded with a mild or none rating. In the coexisting psychopathology group, 60% responded with a mild or none rating. And the classical patients group responded the best with 95% of the patients in this group rating their symptoms as mild or none.

In 1989, Harvey et al.,[3] wondered if the success of the 1987 Whorwell et al., study was dependent upon the abilities of an individual hypnotherapist. To investigate this possibility, they designed a study using two different hypnotherapists in the treatment of refractory IBS. The study involved 33 refractory IBS patients and it also compared group hypnotherapy with individual treatment.

The treatment protocol was the same as the one used in earlier studies, except the patients received ONLY five 40-minute sessions with decreasing frequency over a five-month period.

A combined scale rating the amount of abdominal distension, abdominal pain, and bowel symptoms was used. At the end of the study, no noteworthy differences were found between the patients that had received one-on-one hypnotherapy or group hypnotherapy.

In this study using ONLY five sessions, the results were much different than Whorwell's studies, with only 60% of the patient improving. The actual numbers showed that 13 patients (39.4%) showed no improvement, 9 patients (27.3%) had fewer symptoms and 11 patients (33.3%) were symptom-free. No major differences were found in the response rate between hypnotherapists, men, women, or patients treated one-on-one or in groups. From this study, hypnotherapy in groups with up to eight patients was shown to be as effective as individual therapy.

As you'll notice from the other studies, one of the possible reasons for having only a 60% success rate may have been that ONLY five sessions were used, and the time frame was extended to five months. Studies have shown that patients achieve better ongoing and long-term relief with more than five hypnosis sessions. Some patients may notice substantial symptom relief after only a couple of sessions; however, these patients may notice a gradual return of their symptoms because IBS symptoms are cyclical in nature. Frequent multiple sessions need to be spaced over a period of three to four months. So from this study we have learned that the more sessions the patients have, the better the results. Later studies will show that IBS patients following this multi-session protocol have uninterrupted symptom relief for more than six years after the sessions ended.

Palsson uses a protocol that basically removes the possible problem of needing a "skilled" hypnotherapist. In 1998, Palsson designed a "standardized" seven-session hypnosis protocol to address the problems of IBS. Each of the hypnosis sessions were designed so that "anyone" could verbally delivery the scripts.

The seven scripts are all mainly the same configuration. The scripts include an eye fixation induction and usually include progressive relaxation, a deepening technique (such as counting from one to twenty as the patient imagines going down a staircase or elevator), after which visualizations are given and suggestions are made. The therapist reads the script verbatim to the patient during each session.

During each session, suggestions that the patient is becoming less sensitive to discomfort and pain, and that their bowel sensations no longer bother them are given. These suggestions are directed towards relieving discomfort and pain in the stomach and intestines.

One of the suggestions to accomplish this might be to have the patient visualize a protective coating on their stomach and intestines. Or using a metaphor that has the patient imagine being inside a log cabin and being protected from the ice and wind that is outside, in the same way they are protected from stomach discomfort or pain. To reduce anxiety, the patient might be asked to imagine a garden or a place in nature, or their favorite place where they are free of any cares or troubles. A recording is given to patients after the second session that has suggestions of the body continuing to learn how to increase this sense of comfort and well-being inside.

It is known that psychological distress (anxiety, helplessness, feeling out of control, etc.) may exacerbate IBS symptoms, so visualizing calm relaxing places (like the garden or the patient's favorite place) is part of Palsson's therapy, which could reduce anxiety. No other psychological issues such as depression are addressed.

In 1996, 50 IBS patients were studied by Houghton et al.,[4] in an attempt to quantify the impact of hypnotherapy on their symptoms as well as their quality of life and economic functioning.

The study divided the patients into two groups, one receiving hypnotherapy and the other acting as a control group. A quality of life questionnaire including questions on symptoms, employment, and health seeking behavior was given out to each group. The hypnotherapy group consisted of 25 patients, aged 25 to 55 years (four males and twenty-one females). The control group consisted of 25 patients of comparable IBS severity, aged 21 to 58 years (two males and twenty-three females).

The results of the study showed that IBS patients in the hypnotherapy group had less severe abdominal pain, backache, bloating, bowel habit, flatulence, lethargy, nausea, urinary symptoms, and painful sexual intercourse compared with the control group.

The results of the study also showed that quality of life, such as emotional and physical well-being, mood, and work attitude were also better in the hypnotherapy group compared to the control group. Related to employment, the study showed that the control group took more time off work (79% compared to the hypnotherapy groups 32%). Also the control group visited their general practitioner more often than the hypnotherapy group (58% compared to 21%). Further, none of the six patients who were out of work resumed employment in the control group. Three of the four hypnotherapy patients who were out of work resumed employment.

This study has shown that not only does hypnotherapy relieve IBS symptoms, but it also greatly improves the patient's quality of life and reduces absenteeism from work.

In two studies, Palsson, Burnett, Meyer and Whitehead[5], investigated the possible physiological and psychological means by which hypnotherapy works with patients with severe IBS. In both studies, the therapists read identical hypnosis scripts.

In their first study in 1997, they evaluated the effects on rectal pain thresholds and smooth muscle tone with a barostat before and after treatment. Eighteen patients received seven biweekly hypnosis sessions and used a shorter session audio recording at home between sessions. Even though after treatment the gut-pain thresholds and muscle tension remained unchanged (the same as in the Manchester study), seventeen of the eighteen patients showed significant improvement in their IBS symptoms.

In the second study in 2000, Palsson, Turner, and Johnson[6] used the same treatment protocol (seven biweekly hypnosis sessions) with 24 patients. In this study they also measured changes in blood pressure, finger temperature, forehead electromyographic activity (electromyography is a technique for evaluating and recording the electrical activity produced by skeletal muscles), heart rate, and skin conductance. Levels of anxiety, depression and somatization (psychological distress in the form of somatic symptoms, such as complaints about pain and GI symptoms), were also measured.

As in the first study, no changes in the physical measurements were evident after treatment; however, 21 of the 24 patients showed improvement in not only their IBS symptoms, but in their psychological well-being as well.

The conclusion from these two studies seems to be that hypnosis reduces psychological distress and somatization, and these improvements are unrelated to changes in the physiological parameters measured.

In 1998, Galovski and Blanchard[7] attempted to replicate Whorwell's et al., original 1984 study, but this time using 12 hypnotherapy sessions (the original study used seven half-hour sessions). The 12 IBS sufferers were divided equally into one group that received a 12-week course of hypnotherapy (30 minutes per week), and another symptom monitoring control group. The treatment protocol was the same as the Manchester protocol (except the number of sessions and the time frame were different).

At the end of six weeks, 80% of the patients in the hypnotherapy group were clinically improved, and none of the six patients in the control group had improved. Since after six weeks there was no improvement in the control group, Galovski and Blanchard decided to treat the control group using hypnotherapy. Once the original control group started receiving hypnotherapy, 67% of these "new" patients also reached clinically significant improvement.

In 2002, a study involving 42 patients was carried out by Palsson et al.[8] Seven 45-minute sessions of individual hypnotherapy were completed roughly every other week for 12 weeks. The hypnotherapy sessions were standardized scripts based mainly on the Manchester model.

Significant symptom improvement was seen in the hypnotherapy group, and there was no improvement seen in the control group. The hypnotherapy group provided a global rating of symptom status ten months after treatment. The mean degree of improvement in IBS symptoms compared with pretreatment levels was 68%.

In 2002, continuing investigation in the United Kingdom by Gonsalkorale, Houghton and Whorwell[9] was carried out by practitioners at the hypnotherapy unit of the University Hospital of South Manchester. In this very large study, 250 patients (aged 19 to 79 years) that had IBS for a minimum of two years and were refractory to previous treatment were selected. A control group was not incorporated in this study because previous studies had already established that hypnotherapy was superior to placebo or non-treatment.

During the first visit and at the end of the twelve sessions, questionnaires to measure the severity of the patient's IBS symptoms (such as bowel and extracolonic symptoms) and psychological status (such as anxiety, depression and quality of life) were filled out by the patients. Twelve weekly sessions over a period of three months, plus daily home practice between sessions were used. Therapy sessions were customized according to the patient's needs. After the final session patients were asked to contact the unit if any "flare-ups" occurred.

The success of the study was measured immediately after the last session, and 71% of patients considered their symptoms "very much better" or "moderately better." These patients reported a significant reduction of abdominal pain and bloating and they had fewer disturbances in their bowel habit. Also their extra-colonic score, which includes backaches, body aches, excessive wind, headaches, heartburn, lethargy, nausea, thigh pain, urinary symptoms, and vomiting, were all improved. Anxiety and depression was reduced and quality of life was improved in all sub-groups. The only sub-group where these improvements were not universal was with males with IBS-D (diarrhea-predominant). This sub-group improved far less than the other participants for no known reason.

The previous study by Gonsalkorale et al., (2002) confirmed the beneficial effects of hypnotherapy in a large number of patients but remember results were only measured immediately after the completion of the twelve hypnotherapy sessions, and no long-term follow-up was planned because of complexity in following the large number of patients.

In 2003, Gonsalkorale et al.,[10] decided to follow-up on the previous patients to ascertain the longer-term effects of therapy in terms of symptoms improvement and use of medication. Of the 250 IBS patients in the 2002 study, 204 patients were tracked down and investigated. Of the patients initially responding to treatment, 81% maintained their improvement one to six years after treatment. The remaining 19%, who had only slight or no improvement with hypnotherapy, had little or no change in the follow-up period.

OK, it looks like hypnotherapy does greatly reduce IBS symptoms, but does it work for people who have been suffering for years? Although this is only one case, this study by Galovski and Blanchard[11] demonstrates the value of hypnotherapy even with a patient who had suffered with IBS symptoms for more than 30 years. This patient suffered from refractory IBS and Generalized Anxiety Disorder (GAD). The patient had unsuccessfully tried numerous traditional and non-traditional psychological treatments.

Galovski and Blanchard used hypnotherapy directed primarily at the patient's IBS symptoms. After six treatment sessions using hypnosis, the patient's IBS symptoms had improved by 53%, at which point he stopped individual hypnotherapy treatment and continued autohypnosis with the aid of audiotapes provided by his therapist. Remember we have seen from previous studies that at least seven sessions seems to be required to achieve long-lasting results from gut-directed hypnotherapy.

At the six-month follow-up, continued improvement (70%) was reported by the patient, and the two-year follow-up showed an improvement of 38% in his IBS symptoms.

The subject's levels of depression, as measured by the Beck Depression Inventory, decreased from a pre-treatment score of 13 to 10 at the six-month follow-up, and dropped to 6 at the two-year follow-up.

The subject's levels of anxiety, as measured by the State Trait Anxiety Inventory, had decreased from a pre-treatment score of 49 to 38 at the six-month follow-up, and dropped slightly to 36 at the two-year follow-up. The hypnotherapy treatment also allowed him to substantially decrease his medications.

A study designed by Houghton et al.,[12] in 2002, composed of 20 patients (17 women, and 3 men, aged 17 to 64), investigated emotional effects on visceral sensitivity.

The patients were grouped into the following four categories:

1. Waking state (control group)

2. Hypnosis with induced anger

3. Hypnosis with induced happiness

4. Hypnosis with suggestions of relaxation (neutral emotion)

All patients were studied under fasting conditions and the visceral sensitivity readings were taken at the same time each day. Sensory responses to balloon distension of the rectum were also assessed.

Prior to the hypnosis, in order to induce anger or happiness, patients were asked which sort of situations might produce the required emotional response. During hypnosis, direct suggestions were given to bring about the proper emotion, and in the case of anger, patients were given relaxation and ego strengthening by the end of the session.

The results of the study were as follows:

1. Anger made it easier to cause symptoms, such as discomfort, or urgency, or the desire to defecate.

2. Happiness appeared to have little effect when compared with relaxation or the waking state.

3. Hypnotic relaxation made it more difficult to cause symptoms.

This study confirms the point of view that emotions are involved in visceral hypersensitivity and the perception of symptoms. The study also demonstrates that relaxation is important in reducing IBS symptoms.

In 2004, Gonsalkorale, Toner and Whorwell[13] designed a study to determine whether the improvement in treating IBS with hypnotherapy was related to cognitive change using a validated scale specifically developed for use in such patients.

A total of 78 IBS patients were given twelve hypnotherapy sessions over a three month period. Before beginning the sessions and after the twelve sessions were completed, the patients completed questionnaires (the Hospital Anxiety and Depression Scale and the Cognitive Scale for Functional Bowel Disorders) to measure severity of IBS symptoms, extra-colonic features and psychological status as well as IBS-related cognitions.

The Cognitive Scale for Functional Bowel Disorders measured the IBS-related cognitions. This scale is subdivided into themes relating to bowel function and personal characteristics relevant to IBS that were derived from the typical thoughts of IBS patients.

The study results held up the conclusions shown in previous research, that is, that hypnotherapy not only reduced both IBS symptoms and associated extra-colonic manifestations, but it also improved the patient's quality of life and psychological well-being. More specifically the study showed IBS symptom improvement.

I at least wanted to cover a study related to emotions and IBS, because strong evidence exists that IBS has an important psychological component.

In a 1998, a study was done by Bennett et al.,[14] with 188 outpatients (135 women) that had various functional gastrointestinal disorders (FGID). All patients were less than 70 years of age, and had no difficulty conversing in English. All patients completed psychological and symptom questionnaires. Bennett et al., found a major association between IBS, somatic symptoms, and severity of emotional distress such as anger, anxiety, depression, and goal frustration. Two-thirds of IBS patients had experienced a severe social stress before the start of their abdominal symptoms. Emotional distress was solidly linked to the overall severity and extent of functional gut disturbance, with 98% of patients having been exposed to at least one chronic social stressor for more than a year. The study also revealed a relationship between inadequate emotional support, increasing age, and IBS.

With that understanding of all the previous studies, let's bring the research a little bit more up to date. In 2006, Wilson, Maddison, Roberts, Greenfield, and Singh[15], did a meta-analysis of the effectiveness of hypnotherapy treatments for IBS sufferers. A meta-analysis is created by combining several clinical trials to identify patterns and obtain a better understanding of the effectiveness of the treatment. Wilson et al., reviewed 20 studies and their findings showed positive patient outcomes in hypnotherapy treatments, especially related to long-lasting symptom remission and overall patient-reported well-being. The meta-analysis showed that not only was the intensity of pain reduced, but the patient's frequency of pain had reduced significantly also. It is felt that the use of "gut-specific imagery" is what was able to produce specific symptom improvements.

That's a lot of data for you to take in, so in the next chapter I'll help out and quickly summarize the results of these studies.

24

GUT-DIRECTED HYPNOSIS
TREATMENT SUMMARY

The effectiveness of gut-specific imagery is compelling, and convincing evidence continues to accumulate demonstrating the effectiveness of hypnotherapy (especially gut-directed hypnotherapy) for the effective management of Irritable Bowel Syndrome. Overall, the reports to date may be briefly summarized as follows:

1. Abdominal pain is common in IBS sufferers; therefore, any treatment should include analgesic techniques.

2. Treatment should not only have limited (or no) side effects, but it should also provide both short-term benefits, such as relief from constipation and diarrhea as well as long-term benefits, such as an improved sense of well-being.

3. All major IBS symptoms (abdominal discomfort, abdominal pain, bloating, constipation, and diarrhea) were mild or absent without medication from using gut-directed hypnotherapy.

4. Symptom scores remain relatively constant between those who had completed hypnotherapy more than 5 years ago compared to those who had finished treatment 1 year ago.

5. Reported success rates in ALL studies with any significant number of patients vary from approximately 70% to 90%.

6. Besides the improvement in physical symptoms, hypnotic treatment usually improves psychological well-being and a person's quality of life.

---

7. IBS research suggests that comprehensive treatment should address both physiological symptoms as well as psychological issues.

By now your expectations should be properly set so that it is obvious that if you want to reduce (or even possibly eliminate) your IBS symptoms, then you should find a hypnotherapist that is skilled at using gut-directed hypnotherapy based mainly on the Manchester model. But how would you know if they are skilled in using hypnotherapy for the treatment of IBS?

To help you in determining if a hypnotherapist is skilled in using gut-directed hypnotherapy based mainly on the Manchester model, the next chapter breaks down and details what should be covered during each session. Remember you should **always** be given a quality recording to listen to on a daily basis between sessions.

25

WHAT IS THE TYPICAL PROTOCOL FOR GUT-DIRECTED HYPNOTHERAPY?

Research for over 30 years by Peter Whorwell, Professor of Medicine and Gastroenterology in the University's Medical School and Director of the South Manchester Functional Bowel Service, has shown that gut-directed hypnosis reduces all the symptoms of IBS, whereas drugs, (when they do work) reduce only a few.

The main focus of gut-directed hypnotherapy is to reduce and even eliminate the symptoms of IBS. Many published research studies have verified that hypnosis is effective in treating IBS. Typically, these research studies consist of somewhere between four to twelve sessions. Studies that had five or fewer sessions proved ineffective, whereas, hypnotic treatment with seven or more sessions prove to be very effective. Hypnosis sessions are conducted weekly or once every other week, and usually last around 30 to 60 minutes.

The Manchester Model is well documented. The original 1984 study consisted of seven half-hour sessions of decreasing frequency over a three month period. The same therapist is used throughout all sessions and each of the sessions is done on a one-to-one basis. This model has been highly effective in the treatment and management of IBS, so much so that it has now become the standard approach for the treatment of IBS in England.

Based on the Manchester Model, an overview of the hypnotic treatment of IBS shows the involvement of the following components:

1. First visit includes the patient's personal history, an explanation of hypnosis, and reassurance of its effectiveness and safety.

2. Progressive muscle relaxation (or other relaxation techniques).

3. Deepening techniques.

4. Special place imagery.

5. Use of an anchoring word, such as "calm," or "relax."

6. Ego strengthening.

7. Metaphors (such as the tree or the river metaphor).

8. Gut-directed hypnotherapy.

9. Systematic desensitization in which patient rehearses previously avoided behaviors.

Most gut-directed hypnotherapy protocols use an approach built on the 1984 Manchester hypnotherapy protocol. So let's take a more detailed look into a "typical" protocol.

One of the "keys" to using twelve weekly sessions is the time period (about three months). Other successful gut-directed hypnotherapy protocols use seven sessions spaced two weeks apart (about three and a half months). You might remember from the Harvey et al., study, that five sessions especially spaced over a five month period) was not enough to have short-term or long-term success.

The first visit includes an assessment of the patient's medical and psychological history, as well as a discussion of the seriousness of their current symptoms. During the initial consultation (the intake), there is also a review of past treatments and conclusions of any medical evaluation and tests. Remember IBS is a diagnosis of exclusion and the patient must be medically evaluated to make a definite diagnosis that they have IBS.

As in any hypnotherapy session, during the first session rapport is established. One of the first session's objectives is also to familiarize the patient with hypnosis and the treatment setting. An explanation of hypnosis is given, including what hypnosis is and especially what hypnosis is NOT is also explained. Reassurance of the effectiveness and safety of hypnosis is also discussed.

Also during the intake, the origin of the patient's symptoms is explained, based on the concept of abnormal gut sensitivity and muscle spasms. Realistic expectations are set concerning length of treatment and when the patient should expect to notice an improvement. Typically, a patient will notice a marked improvement by the fourth hypnotherapy session.

At this point the patient is given a symptom log sheet to record their IBS symptoms daily in detail. The daily symptom log usually contains the date, and a list of symptoms, such as bloating, constipation, diarrhea, gas, stool consistency, and pain. There may also be a column for diet, medications, supplements, and vitamins.

All sessions include a hypnotic induction, and progressive relaxation is typically used during the first session. This allows the patient to experience what hypnosis feels like first-hand. Progressive relaxation as an induction takes some time, so this session is usually one of the longest. A recording (CD, Mp3, etc.) is sent home with the patient to be listened to daily. This sets the expectation with the patient that to be successful with this program the recording must be listened to on a daily basis. The patient MUST be committed to listening to the recording on a daily basis to reinforce the treatment. The importance of this cannot be over-stressed. The first recording lasts about 30 minutes and is relaxing, but it does not typically contain any gut-directed suggestions.

In the protocol that I use, I prefer to have the second session in the week following the initial session, although sometimes the second visit is scheduled two weeks after the first one. This allows for a baseline of the patient's symptoms to be recorded. The hypnotherapy sessions are optimally scheduled no more than two weeks apart until the entire sequence is completed.

The following is an overview of the gut-directed hypnosis protocol that I use:

1. Induction (eye-fixation, progressive relaxation, autogenics, favorite place, etc.).

2. Trance-deepening (counting down, going down stairs, going down in an escalator or elevator, sinking down on a cloud, etc.).

3. Special place or "therapeutic scene" imagery using multiple senses and metaphors (such as the tree or the river metaphor). This allows the patient to dissociate and increases relaxation.

4. Therapeutic suggestions including gut-directed hypnotherapy.

5. Confidence-building, ego strengthening, and general suggestions for well-being.

6. Post-hypnotic suggestions.

7. Future pacing to "practice" new behaviors.

8. Trance termination.

The hypnotherapy protocol for IBS follows the basic protocol for any hypnotherapy session. The patient is "relaxed" in some way (induction), and then trance-deepening techniques are used. After this, different therapeutic modules (suggestions) or metaphors are used. Suggestions, (gut-directed suggestions for IBS patients), are always after trance-deepening so that the patient is in a receptive state. In this way, therapeutic suggestions for change can be accepted. Ego strengthening and post-hypnotic suggestions are used. Future pacing helps the patient envision their life after their problems (or symptoms) have significantly changed. And of course trance termination ends the hypnosis part of the session.

OK, you now have a good overview of the gut-directed hypnosis session protocol, so let's go a little bit more in depth.

All hypnotic techniques use a hypnotic induction. Progressive muscle relaxation is one technique; however, this technique takes the most time to carry out. There is an active progressive relaxation where the patient tenses their muscles above their normal tension level, and then releases the tension. There is also passive progressive relaxation. Passive relaxation doesn't require the patient to tense their muscles. There are many other induction techniques, and some are covered in the chapter called, "What are the Current Strategies for Treating IBS?"

One of the techniques used during the hypnotic induction is to have the patient focus on their breathing while silently repeating a key word, such as calm or relax. This technique usually slows down the pace of the patient's breathing, which improves relaxation. Also the word calm or relax encourages a sense of internal peace and tranquility.

"Take a moment and picture and imagine that with every breath you take in, a little bit more calm enters your body. Breathing in pure relaxation ... (the ... means pause for a second or two) and breathing out any tension or worry ... Slowly, comfortably, each cell of your body begins to experience a new found calmness."

Trance-deepening is the process of making a trance state more intense. The goal of deepening is to make sure that the unconscious mind will be more accepting of suggestion. You don't want your conscious mind analyzing everything that is said.

Deepening can be done by counting down, such as:

"In a moment, I'm going to count down from 10 to 1. With each number you hear, allow your relaxation to double, as you drift down deeper into the tranquil stillness of your mind."

Breathing can also be counted, such as:

"Allow each easy and natural breathe you take to bring you a little bit deeper into relaxation. One ... breathing in comfort ..."

Hypnosis deepening by visualization is done by constructing pictures in your mind. These places can be real or imagined. It's important to be looking through your own eyes when visualizing so that you are associated to the experience. You want the feeling of being there and the experience of it happening to you now.

Places that you relate with relaxation and peace of mind work really well. You might be lying on a chase-lounge in the filtered sunlight on a golden sanded beach listening to the sound of the waves. Or maybe you prefer walking down a country path and smelling the beautiful wildflowers on a clear summer's day. Or maybe being in the mountains at a healing spa overlooking a gently flowing river is relaxing for you.

Deepening can be done by combining visualization with counting, such as:

"Picture and imagine that you are standing at the top of a beautiful set of ten stairs. The steps are very wide, and very safe, and of your favorite color and material. With each number you hear, and with each step you take down, allow

yourself to go deeper into relaxation. Let's start now by taking the first step down to step 9 and simply relaxing ... 8 ... more and more deeply relaxed with each step you take ... 7 ... going even deeper now ... 6 ... etc."

Using an escalator or an elevator works in a similar fashion:

"I want you to find yourself standing in front of an elevator that has five floors. In a moment I'm going to ask you to step into the elevator and push the button for the bottom floor. As the elevator descends, allow yourself to go deeper into relaxation. And when you reach the bottom floor and step off of the elevator, you will step into a deep state of relaxation ... deeper than you've ever felt before. OK, let's get started. Step into the elevator, push the button for the bottom floor, and watch as the doors quietly close. As you feel the elevator start to smoothly go down, you descend with it, floor after floor, and drift deeper into relaxation. Effortlessly moving towards the bottom floor and feeling even more relaxed. You're getting closer to that place that brings wonderful feelings of tranquility to your body and peace to your mind (etc)."

Deepening can also be done by direct suggestion, such as:

"Each time you listen to this recording you will go into an even deeper state of relaxation."

Or how about:

"With each breath you take you find yourself relaxing just that much more and going even deeper ... even deeper still."

After deepening, special places, therapeutic scenes, or metaphors are used, allowing the patient to further dissociate and relax.

Some scenes might include a journey through the digestive system, or a protection metaphor, such as imagining remaining comfortable inside a mountain cabin on a stormy night. You might be asked to imagine that no matter what is happening inside or outside the cabin … you continue to feel warm, safe, and protected.

Each session might use a different special place, therapeutic scene, or metaphor. A tree metaphor might be used where the unconscious mind is the root of all knowledge, resources, and strengths. A tree is also flexible and bends with the conditions outside. Leaves falling off the tree might represent all anxiety, doubts, and worries falling away.

The river metaphor has been successfully used in the treatment of IBS within the UK National Health Service (Whorwell, 2006)[1, 2]and in single case studies.[3, 4, 5] For those patients suffering from IBS-D (diarrhea), the river metaphor directs the patient's attention to a fast flowing river, and the patient is given the chance to alter the image so that the river narrows down to a slower-paced smooth flowing stream. In the case of patients with IBS-C (constipation), the metaphor of a blocked-up river is utilized and the patient is directed to remove the debris and obstacles so that the stream runs smoothly. A gatekeeper could also control the gates to the river. This gives the patient control over the speed of the river and therefore the patient can adjust the flow of water according to their individual bowel patterns.

The use of the river metaphor serves two purposes. It relates directly to the problems the patient is having with their bowels (constipation or diarrhea) and it directs the patient, at the unconscious level, to review the emotional content of their symptoms. Think for a moment what a tumultuous or blocked river might represent symbolically. Emotional processing of inner conflicts is often a major factor in recovery, and by directing the patient to imagine a smooth flowing river, they can evaluate any emotional conflict, which in turn, can reprogram and restore normal gut activity.

During the therapeutic scene or metaphor, enough time should be given so that the patient can explore the imagery in their own way. In the case of the river metaphor the images used are important, but again it's up to the patient to make the connections that are most appropriate for them so they can gain greater meaning from the imagery.

Trees alongside the river can represent flexibility and strength. A smooth flowing river can represent a normal functioning digestive system. If parts of the river create shimmering pools, then the patient may take some time for "reflection" and examine parts of their life. The patient might also imagine what it would be like to drift and float comfortably down the river on a raft or in a canoe.

To encourage normal bowel functioning, the hypnotherapist could say something like:

"Your bowel movements are returning to a stable healthy natural routine."

You might remember the name Emile Coue (1857–1926) and his comment, "Every day in every way I am getting better and better." Coue was a French psychologist and he felt that by repeating positive suggestions to ones-self that the suggestions would take hold in the person's unconscious mind. Nowadays we might refer to these suggestions as ego strengthening, which was popularized by John Hartland around 1966. Ego strengthening suggestions boost the patient's confidence and self-worth.

Here are some ego strengthening suggestions to increase the IBS sufferer's sense of health and comfort:

1. You are going to feel physically stronger and healthier with each passing day.

2. You deserve and are becoming strong and healthy.

3. Your energy continues to increase.

4. Every day your emotions are much calmer, and you feel much more settled.

5. Your GI tract is returning to normal functioning.

6. Day by day, any external or internal irritations fade away being replaced with a sense of tranquility.

7. Your feelings of personal well-being continue to increase.

Post-hypnotic suggestions are given while the patient is in a state of hypnosis. The suggestions made will help the patient "learn" a new behavior and the suggestions will take place after the hypnotic session has ended. Post-hypnotic suggestions are given to reduce the patient's abdominal pain, and to have them regain control over their bowel function. Audio recordings help to reinforce these suggestions and at-home therapy has been shown to be effective (Gonsalkorale, 2006)[6]; Kearney and Brown-Chang, 2008.[7]

Posthypnotic suggestions usually have the following form:

> "From now on, when/whenever/each time/each and every time X stimulus), you will Y (response)."

For most people, the concept of warmth brings about feelings of comfort, so the patient could be told to place their hand on their abdomen and feel a warming sensation begin to radiate throughout their entire abdomen. This could take the form of:

"Anytime you place your hand on your abdomen, you will enjoy a pleasant warming and soothing sensation."

This suggestion follows the posthypnotic protocol. "Anytime you place your hand on your abdomen," is the stimulus, and, "you will enjoy a pleasant warming and soothing sensation" is the response. So this suggestion acts as a conditioned response, such that any time the patient puts their hand on their abdomen they will feel a sense of warmth and comfort (allowing relief of their symptoms.)

To further reinforce this suggestion, the hypnotherapist could say:

"Each and every time you place your hand on your abdomen ... you feel better ... you feel comfortable ... and you know, really know that your GI tract is returning to normal."

Other post-hypnotic suggestions can be given to gradually reduce the patient's symptoms, such as:

"As each day passes, that old discomfort continues to diminish, which means that ... you have more control over your GI tract."

During the hypnotic process, many direct and indirect suggestions are used to suggest to the patient that their symptoms are decreasing, both in frequency and in intensity. Here is an example:

"Those old unpleasant feelings continue to diminish, because you now tend to focus on what you want in life."

New skills can also be suggested:

"Day by day, your ability to manage your GI symptoms improve, because like any new skill, the more you practice the more your ability improves."

Future pacing is a type of mental imagery that is used so that the patient can imagine themselves in the future having a normal GI tract and living a good life. Remember the mind cannot tell the difference between something that is "real" and something that is vividly imagined. The idea of future pacing is to have the patient see themselves already having achieved the desired change.

"I want you to go out one month or three months or six months and picture, imagine, and really feel what it's like having a normal GI system and living a normal life. That old abdominal pain has faded away, and your bowel habits are now quite predictable."

After about 30 to 40 minutes of being in hypnosis, it's time to end the hypnosis session and bring the patient out of trance and back into normal awareness. This is typically done by counting the patient back up. A simple way to do this is as follows:

"In a moment I'm going to count from one to five. When I reach the count of five, you will be totally out of the hypnotic state. One ..."

At the end of each hypnotherapy session, the patient is given a (hypnotic) recording containing suggestions for relaxation, as well as gut-directed suggestions, for daily home use.

That's a lot of data to take in, so let's take a moment to let it sink in ... OK the moment's up! Let's look at the objective of gut-directed hypnotherapy and what should occur during each hypnotherapy session.

26

WHAT CAN YOU
EXPECT IN EACH
IBS HYPNOTHERAPY SESSION?

You now know what should be included during the typical protocol for gut-directed hypnotherapy. Remember, the main focus of gut-directed hypnotherapy is to reduce and even eliminate the symptoms of IBS. Hypnotherapy provides significant short-term relief and long-lasting improvement in bowel symptoms with improved psychological well-being.

Now let's break-down the typical gut-directed hypnotherapy treatments by session.

I already described the purpose of the first visit. It's all about assessing the patient's medical and psychological history, and reviewing past treatments and conclusions of any medical evaluation and tests. Rapport is established, and a discussion about what hypnosis is and is NOT is explained. Realistic expectations are set, and a symptom log sheet is given to the patient.

The second session usually includes a simpler hypnotic induction, deepening techniques, and more specific techniques aimed at controlling and normalizing gut function are introduced (such as a journey through the digestive system), and again, suggestions for general confidence-building, ego-strengthening and increased well-being are given.

Suggestions for tapping into the unconscious mind's ability to control gut function are usually given in the second or third session. This could take the form of:

"Picture and imagine that you are in the control room of your mind. Take a moment and find the dial that controls abdominal pain. Notice where the dial is currently set, and slowly turn the setting down so that ... your abdomen feels more comfortable."

Other suggestions similar to the one above can be used to direct and gain more control over the patient's GI tract.

The remaining sessions are similar to the second session. The inductions are kept simple because by now the patient is used to drifting off into a hypnotic state. If they have been listening to the recordings on a daily basis, then they will have been "hypnotized" about 21 times (three weeks). The patient will be more likely to listen to shorter recordings, so this is another reason that a simple induction is used.

From the third session onwards, after an induction and deepening techniques have been used, hypnotic suggestions intended to normalize GI function are given. The suggestions given include some or all of the following:

1. Direct and indirect suggestions for relaxation

2. Guided imagery to deepen overall physical relaxation

3. Gut-directed suggestions for normalizing the GI function

4. Suggestions for reducing gut discomfort (possibly inducing a sense of comfort, specifically comfort in the abdomen)

5. Age regression techniques

6. Suggestions for confidence improvement

7. Suggestions for general well-being

8. Suggestions for creating a protective shield

Patients are also expected to listen to their audio recording daily.

At the end of the third session, the patient is again given a symptom log sheet to record their IBS symptoms daily in detail for the next two weeks. They will bring this log with them to the fourth session. This gives both the hypnotherapist and the patient a good comparison of how they are progressing.

Once the seven to twelve session sequence has come to an end (which typically takes about three plus months), the therapy course is completed and generally no further treatment is necessary. For most patients (80% or more) their IBS symptoms have disappeared or they know that they are putting themselves in a stressful situation and they will take the necessary precautions to improve their well-being.

After the last session, a "maintenance" recording is given to the patient. This recording acts as a booster session and is only used when needed. In some cases, a follow-up session will be scheduled about one to three months after the last session. In general, most patient's bowel symptoms continue to improve in the months after completing the typical gut-directed hypnotherapy protocol.

We have covered a lot of ground, so you are probably wondering (and it's OK to wonder), what conclusions related to treating IBS can be drawn about diet, medications, alternative treatments, imagery in healing, mind-body communication, and especially gut-directed hypnotherapy. Let's look at those conclusions.

27

CONCLUSIONS

This book highlights the use of hypnotherapy as a treatment for IBS, and has provided a good review of hypnosis studies since 1984. The results of these studies confirm that gut-directed hypnotherapy is an effective treatment for refractory IBS. And yet in spite of the remarkable results, hypnosis for the treatment of IBS is not widely available, or even widely known about.

Because most IBS suffers do not notice much improvement (even with good medical care) from standard medical treatment, other alternative methods have been sought after. Gut-directed hypnotherapy is an important treatment alternative to the standard medical treatment that uses changes in diet, and medications to manage IBS symptoms. Gut-directed hypnotherapy treatment works even if the IBS patient has not received any benefit from medications or other regular medical treatments.

Hypnotherapy helps at least three out of every four patients who have not improved from standard medical treatment to gain substantial and long-lasting bowel symptom relief. Remember, standard medical treatment helps about one out of every four patients.

Current pharmacological treatment focuses on treating individual IBS symptoms such as abdominal pain, constipation, and diarrhea. The scientific data shows that the effectiveness of these drugs in the treatment of IBS is inadequate at best[1]. Pharmacological treatments have potential side-effects and are expensive.

Gut-directed hypnotherapy does not have any of the side-effects associated with pharmacological treatments. Hypnotherapy reduces abdominal pain, bloating, and distention. Constipation and diarrhea are also improved through hypnotherapy treatment. There is about a 70% to 90% probability of significant improvement in IBS symptoms and overall well-being, and for most people, this improvement lasts for years without any further treatment. The gut-directed hypnotherapy protocol is highly reproducible, and both short-term and long-term symptom improvements occur.

Long-term improvements have been demonstrated to last beyond two years, and the vast majority of patients maintain these improvements for more than five years. With all these positive results, I'm sure that you would agree that a case for using hypnotherapy in the treatment of IBS can be easily made. Gut-directed hypnotherapy is most likely more effective than any other single treatment modality for moderate to severe IBS.

Even though hypnotherapy can make a major difference in a patient's life, it must be noted that it is not to be considered a cure for IBS. There is no assurance that a patient's symptoms will never reoccur. Now and then an extra session of hypnotherapy may be required. One of the advantages of hypnotherapy is that it puts the patient back in control of their life again.

Besides the effects on GI symptoms, there are positive effects related to the patient's quality of life. Hypnotherapy brings about a reduction in depression and a significant reduction in anxiety. Besides having long-lasting effects, hypnotherapy as an intervention has a high degree of patient satisfaction.

There is no one ideal treatment for IBS because IBS patients present with a mixed degree of symptoms which have varying regularities and severities. The majority of IBS patients (around 70%), have mild symptoms and infrequently consult their primary care providers. This group lives a relatively normal life; however, times of stress tend to cause their symptoms to flare-up. This group also has little or no psychosocial difficulties and typically no psychological treatments are required. In the conventional medical system, their treatment usually centers on diet and medications, with a little bit of education and reassurance thrown in.

The next IBS group has moderate symptoms (about 25%). Their symptoms are typically irregular, and every so often can be so severe that the patient becomes socially and emotionally disabled. Current medical treatments utilize pharmacological drugs that have a host of side-effects and again have been shown to be less than effective.

The remaining 5% of IBS patients have severe symptoms, including constant pain, anxiety, and depression. They may have a history of sexual or physical abuse, and because there is no effective treatment, they tend to use the health care system a lot more than the other 95% of IBS sufferers.

In patients that have either moderate or severe symptoms, it is a well-known fact that if the patient does not already have some type of psychiatric disorder, they soon will. Over the years this has been thoroughly studied, and the results show that patients with IBS have a higher prevalence of primarily psychiatric disorders compared to the general population. In female IBS sufferers these numbers can run as high as 50%[2].

The next chapter will assist you in finding a hypnotherapist that understands IBS and how to treat it.

28

OK, MY EXPECTATIONS ARE SET! NOW WHAT DO I DO?

The difficulty with using hypnotherapy to reduce or eliminate IBS symptoms is not with the protocol; the protocol works! The challenge is that you will need to find a hypnotherapist who understands IBS and is an expert in gut-directed hypnotherapy.

Currently hypnosis is not restricted or regulated by law in many states in the US, and there are also no government regulations in the UK. As with any form of treatment, it is important to find a practitioner who is qualified and well-trained.

Some professionals will insist that you find a person who is a state-licensed health professional, such as a psychologist, nurse, physician, or clinical social worker who knows the hypnotherapy protocol for IBS. I have a slightly different opinion about who may be best qualified to provide treatment for your IBS symptoms.

Let's start at the beginning. To assist the IBS patient in returning to a higher quality of life two things must happen: a diagnosis must be made, and a comprehensive treatment plan must be put in place.

You **DO** need a physician (probably a gastroenterologist is your best choice) to run the required tests to diagnosis you with IBS. But think about this for a moment, IBS is a diagnosis of exclusion, which means that lots of tests will need to be run to rule out other diseases. After your physician rules out any other disease, which means that they can find no identifiable structural or biochemical cause, such as inflammation, or infection, or structural abnormality, then if the patient meets the Rome III criteria, your physician can make a diagnosis and label it as Irritable Bowel Syndrome.

OK, a diagnosis of IBS has been made, so the next step is a comprehensive treatment plan. Almost all (if not all) IBS patients will be told to change their diet and medications will be prescribed. Again, you will want your physician to be recommending and over-seeing this part of your treatment. I'm in complete agreement with standard medical treatment up to this point. At this point we know that 25% of IBS patients will "respond" in some form to this type of treatment. My question is, "Who is the best professional qualified to treat the other 75% using gut-directed hypnotherapy?"

Hypnotizing a person by itself will not help reduce or eliminate a person's IBS symptoms. The benefits of hypnosis occur **after** the hypnotic state has been induced. It is this part of the IBS protocol that requires specialized hypnotic knowledge and training.

Hypnosis may be the treatment of choice, especially when severe chronic symptoms continue after standard medical management approaches are not providing adequate relief. Remember, treatment using gut-directed hypnotherapy can produce improvement that lasts for years.

In a few highly specialized gastrointestinal centers, hypnotherapy is already used to treat patients that have IBS. So if you're near Whorwell's center in England, I would suggest that you go there, or if you're able to get some help from the UNC Center for Functional GI and Motility Disorders in North Carolina at Chapel Hill, well that's a good choice also. But what if you're not near England or North Carolina in the United States? What do you do then?

My opinion is that you find a hypnotherapist that knows the gut-directed protocol created by the Manchester group. Whorwell acknowledges that it's essential to find a hypnotherapist who knows what he/she is doing ... and more importantly ... knows about IBS. You want to find a person who has had formal training and considerable experience in clinical hypnosis, especially in treating IBS. Using hypnosis requires considerable language skills and knowledge, and to successfully treat IBS, specific gut-directed suggestions and imagery need to be included.

It is best if the hypnotherapist has been referred directly by a physician, and your hypnotherapist should ask (you) the patient for a referral from your doctor before any gut-directed hypnotherapy sessions begin. Also, many health insurance plans in the US reimburse for IBS treatment with hypnosis when it is billed as psychological treatment under the mental health portion of the plans. So if your doctor prescribes hypnotherapy you may be covered (check with your insurance carrier for their specific requirements).

If your physician does not work directly with a hypnotherapist that uses gut-directed hypnotherapy, then you can use the information that I have provided in this book on what the protocol is, and what you should expect during each session. Once again, you as a patient are responsible for listening to the various audio recording daily between each face-to-face session with your hypnotherapist.

But what if your physician cannot give you a referral and you cannot find a hypnotherapist in your area that knows gut-directed hypnotherapy? Then what do you do?

Another option is to use gut-directed audio recordings that you can listen to on your own. If you remember from our earlier discussions, studies have been carried out comparing the differences between individual sessions versus group sessions, and recording (audiotape) versus therapist, with the results showing little difference in outcome. Don't get me wrong, when you are sitting face-to-face with a therapist, there will be other "stuff" (consider "stuff" to be a technical term) that comes up. And dealing with this stuff will probably improve the quality of your life.

Listening to gut-directed hypnotherapy recordings are considered as having a relatively high success rate in alleviating IBS symptoms (significantly more than twice as effective as the standard change of diet and medication treatment). The patient must be motivated to follow the at home program on their own, which is no different than the expectation that the patient will listen to the audio recordings daily when they are seeing their hypnotherapist. One advantage of listening to gut-directed hypnotherapy audio recordings is the cost. An entire hypnotherapy audio recording program probably costs less than a single session with a hypnotherapist.

So of course your next question is going to be, "Where do I find quality audio recordings that utilize the Manchester gut-directed hypnotherapy protocol for IBS?" After hearing this question from a number of people, I decided to create the audio recordings that you need. So let's look at the next chapter and see what's in these recordings.

29

WHAT'S IN THE GUT-DIRECTED HYPNOTHERAPY AUDIO RECORDINGS?

I've created a set of audio recordings (CDs) that are similar to the ones I use when working with patients that have been diagnosed with IBS. (The recordings I use are custom, that is, they include the client's name and specific suggestions are added that are unique to the client).

When listening to hypnosis recordings choose an environment that is quiet and safe. Using headphones typically will reduce outside noise; however this is not necessary to become relaxed.

**Never listen to these recordings
while driving a car or operating machinery**

These recordings also use isochronic brainwave entrainment. Brainwave entrainment is considered quite safe but isn't appropriate for everyone. **Those who should avoid brainwave entrainment include the following:** epileptics or anyone prone to seizures; pregnant women; anyone who wears a pacemaker; anyone who is photosensitive; and anyone under the age of 18 (those under the age of 18 are more prone to seizures and quite possibly haven't been diagnosed as of yet). Also, never listen to hypnosis recordings (with or without brainwave entrainment) when under the influence of alcohol or drugs and to say it again, never listen to hypnosis recordings while driving a vehicle or operating machinery. If you are using medication, consult a physician before listening to recordings with brainwave entrainment.

For the best outcome, each of the recordings should be listened to daily according to the schedule that is given to the patient. It is up to you to be an active participant in your healing by listening to these recordings each day.

There are eight sessions; however, there are twelve recordings. You will find that Session 4 has three recordings. One recording is for constipation-predominate IBS (Session 4C), one recording is for diarrhea-predominate IBS (Session 4D), and one recording is for alternating constipation and diarrhea (Session 4M). You should choose the recording that best fits your symptoms. There is also a recording if you have anxiety and another recording if you have depression, which are not at all unusual if you have IBS.

The first recording that you will listen to is the "Listen To First" recording. This recording gives a detailed explanation about the program and brain waves. There is an IBS Symptom Tracking Chart (see the end of this chapter), that you will fill out to track your progress as you listen to each session.

The first session (Session 1) uses progressive relaxation and is ONLY used to get you accustomed to relaxing during a "hypnotic" session. There are no specific gut-directed metaphors or IBS suggestions on this first recording. This recording should be listened to daily for one week before listening to the next recording.

If you have symptoms of anxiety, then I suggest that you listen to the Calm and Relaxed recording after Session 1. You will listen to this recording to reduce your anxiety for a week. If you do NOT have symptoms of depression, THEN you will continue on to Session 2 through Session 8 in that order.

If you also have symptoms of depression, then I suggest that you listen to the Riding the Rapids recording AFTER the anxiety recording. You will listen to this recording for a week, THEN you will continue on to Session 2 through Session 8 in that order.

If you also have symptoms of depression, but do NOT have symptoms of anxiety, then I suggest that you listen to the Riding the Rapids recording AFTER Session 1. You will listen to this recording to reduce your symptoms of depression for a week, THEN you will continue on to Session 2 through Session 8 in that order.

The first session uses progressive relaxation and is used for relaxing, whereas the next recordings, sessions two through eight, use the gut-directed hypnotherapy protocol that has been successfully used with IBS patients for more than 30 years. Each of these sessions, sessions two through eight, should be listened to in order for two-weeks before listening to the next recording. Each of these sessions contain a slightly different induction, deepening, metaphor, and of course various gut-directed suggestions.

You will find that Session 4 has three recordings. One recording is for constipation-predominate IBS (Session 4C), one recording is for diarrhea-predominate IBS (Session 4D), and one recording is for alternating constipation and diarrhea (Session 4M). You should choose the recording that best fits your symptoms. After listening to Session 4, you will continue with Session 5, Session 6, Session 7, and Session 8. Session 8 is your maintenance session.

After finishing listening to Session 2, Session 3, Session 4, and Session 5, most patients notice a definite change for the better in their IBS symptoms. For some people, this change happens sooner, and for other patients noticeable changes take longer to occur.

The final recording, Session 8, is your maintenance recording, and it is the shortest of the recordings. Listen to this recording like you would the other recording, that is, daily for two-weeks. At that point you should only need to listen to the Session 8 maintenance recording on an as needed basis.

If you're wondering why you need to listen to the recordings for a period of time, well it's because IBS symptoms repeat from time to time. This means that it is essential to use numerous hypnotherapy sessions spaced over a period of three to four months to attain long-lasting results.

If you are currently taking medications, then you should continue with your medications until your symptoms have been reduced or eliminated. Once that has happened let your doctor know so that he/she can recommend the appropriate course of action.

IBS Listening Schedule

For the best outcome, these recordings should be listened to daily. It is up to you to be an active participant in your healing by listening to these recordings each day.

If you are NOT listening to the Calm and Relaxed or the Riding the Rapids recording, then the period of time required to listen to all the recordings is as follows:

Session 1 – Daily for 1 week

Session 2 – Daily for 2 weeks

Session 3 – Daily for 2 weeks

Session 4 – Daily for 2 weeks

Session 5 – Daily for 2 weeks

Session 6 – Daily for 2 weeks

Session 7 – Daily for 2 weeks

Session 8 – Daily for 2 weeks

Total period of time is about 15 weeks (again, if you are not listening to either the anxiety or the depression recordings). After that you can listen to your favorite recording on an as needed basis.

It is important that you record the levels of your IBS symptoms on the IBS Symptom Tracking Chart. This is more important than you may think. Studies have shown that whatever you measure improves. So if you want to get the most from this program, then I strongly suggest that you record your symptoms on a daily basis, and if possible do this without looking at the previous day's numbers.

IBS TRACKING CHART SCALE RATING

Rate your symptoms on a scale of 0 to 10	
0	No presenting problems.
Mild 1 - 2	Symptoms hardly ever occur. If present, abdominal pain is minor.
Moderate 3 - 4	Symptoms sometimes interfere with daily life. Abdominal pain is moderate, but controllable.
Strong 5 - 6	Symptoms cause schedule changes more than 50% of the time. Abdominal pain may be strong.
Harsh 7 - 8	Most of the time you are out of action. Abdominal pain is moderate to severe.
Relentless 9 - 10	Incapable of leaving the house (out of action). Abdominal pain is severe to intense.

IBS SYMPTOM TRACKING CHART

Chart Key:

C = Constipation, D = Diarrhea,
F = Fatigue, G = Gas,
AP = Abdominal Pain,
AD = Abdominal Distention,
SC = Stool Consistency,
LTCD = Listened to CD

Date	C	D	F	G	A P	A D	S C	LTCD

HOW DO I
GET THE IBS CDS?

The IBS CDs are available from Amazon. If you are ready to finally reduce or eliminate your IBS symptoms and reclaim your life then go to the following webpage:

http://www.Amazon.com/dp/B0OO0BK70I

Click on Add to Cart

That's it! Now all that's left to do is to wait a couple of days and then enjoy the audio recordings.

Now it's time to learn about the author. Who is this guy, and why did he take all this time to write this comprehensive book on IBS? Well ... let's look at the next chapter and find out.

ABOUT THE AUTHOR

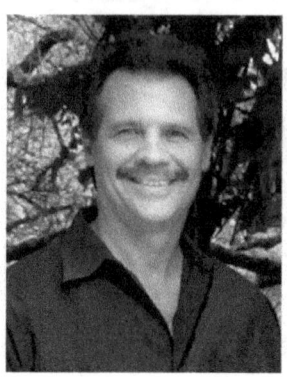

Larry Siebert Ph.D. is one of only a handful of people in this country with a Doctor of Philosophy degree in Clinical Hypnotherapy. Dr. Siebert has been in private practice since 1996 and is a Registered Hypnotherapist, Certified Hypnosis Instructor, and Certified Trainer of Master Time Line Therapy™. He is a Master Practitioner and Certified Trainer of Neuro-Linguistic Programming.

In his previous life, Larry had a successful 25-plus-year career as a hardware design engineer, including designing the circuit boards that are used in computing devices. His natural ability in finding patterns and visualizing pathways uniquely qualified him to design these complex boards that must be able to transmit tens of thousands of instructions along the most efficient and successful routes.

It was with great satisfaction that Larry realized that his abilities also enable him to discover the patterns and pathways in the workings of the minds and emotions of people, and that through

Hypnotherapy, Neuro-Linguistic Programming, and Huna he is able to assist people in discovering their current patterns and change them to more successful and enjoyable ones. If given the right "interface" a person will go from where they are currently to where they want to be.

Larry finds it fascinating to go through the discovery with his clients of how their "wiring" is forming their current expectations and experiences of life. He finds his fulfillment through assisting people in moving past their obstacles and living the lives they desire.

Larry is also a student of the Hawaiian healing and shamanistic science of Huna. He has created many seminars, including Huna Dream Interpretation, Creating Prosperity™, Understanding Your Partner & Yourself, and others that utilize extensive hypnotherapy modalities.

ONE LAST THING

Thank you for purchasing *IBS Gut Instinct*. If you enjoyed this book or found it useful, besides telling everyone, I'd be very grateful if you would be kind and post a short review on Amazon. Your support really does make a difference and I do read ALL the reviews personally so I can get your feedback and make future versions of this book even better.

If you would like to leave a review then all you need to do is go to the following link:

http://www.amazon.com/dp/B00R3UBOPA

(which is the *IBS Gut Instinct* page). Once there, scroll down to the bottom of the Customer Reviews section and find the box labeled "Write a customer review."

When you're done leaving a review take a screenshot of it and email it to me at **drlarry@LarrySiebert.com**

When you do that I'll send you a link to my 10 minute *Simply Relaxed* recording as my special thanks for leaving a review.

If you have any questions about

IBS Gut Instinct,

please contact me at:
drlarry@LarrySiebert.com

Thanks again for your support!

OTHER BOOKS BY
LARRY SIEBERT PH.D.

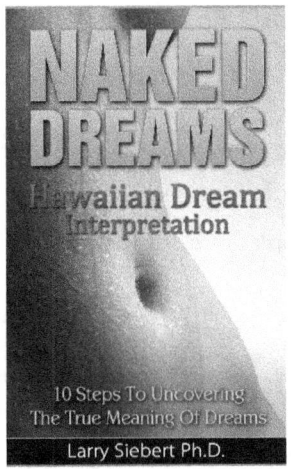

Check out

Naked Dreams

Hawaiian Dream Interpretation

By going to

http://www.amazon.com/dp/B00GVGJJ5E/

34

REFERENCES

What's Different About This Book On IBS?

1. Mearin F, Badia X, Balboa A, Benavent J, Caballero AM, Dominguez-Munoz E, Garrigues V, Pique JM, Roset M, Cucala M, Figueras M: Predictive factors of irritable bowel syndrome improvement: 1-year prospective evaluation in 400 patients. *Aliment Pharmacol Therapy* 2006, 23 (6): 815 – 826.

2. Vliege AM, Rutten J, Govers A, Frankenhuis C, and Benninga MA: Long-Term Follow-Up of Gut-Directed Hypnotherapy vs. Standard Care in Children With Functional Abdominal Pain or Irritable Bowel Syndrome. *American Journal Gastroenterol* 2012; 107:627–631; published online 7 February 2012.

What Is Irritable Bowel Syndrome (IBS)?

1. Lovell RM, Ford AC. Global Prevalence of and Risk Factors for Irritable Bowel Syndrome: A Meta-analysis. *Clinical Gastroenterol Hepatol*, 2012.

Is IBS Really A Problem?

1. Adapted from Camilleris M, et al. *Alimentary Pharmacology Theaputics.* 1997; 11:3.

2. Muller-Lisners et al. *Digestion*, 2001; 64-200.

What Causes IBS?

1. *American Journal of Medicine*, 1989; 86: 262-6.

How Is IBS Diagnosed?

1. Manning AP, Thompson WG, Heaton KW, et al. Towards positive diagnosis of the irritable bowel. *Br Med J* 1978; 2:653–654.

2. Hungin AP, Whorwell PJ, Tack J, Mearin F, The prevalence, patterns and impact of irritable bowel syndrome: An international survey of 40,000 subjects. *Aliment Pharmacol Therapy.* 2003 Mar1: 17(5): 643-50.

What Are The Current Strategies For Treating IBS?

1. Bensoussan A, Talley NJ, Hing M et al. Treatment of irritable bowel syndrome with Chinese herbal medicine: a randomized controlled trial. *Journal of the American Medical Association.* 1998; 280(18): 1585-1589.

2. Leung W.K., Wu JC, Liang Sm, Chan LS, Chan FK, Xie H, Fung SS, Hui AJ, Wong, VM, Che CT, Sung JJ. Treatment of diarrhea-predominate irritable bowel symptom with traditional Chinese herbal medicine: A randomized placebo-controlled trial. *American Journal Gastroenterol* 2006 Jul; 101 (7):1574-80.

3. Blanchard EB,Schwarz SP. Adaptation of a multicomponent treatment for irritable bowel syndrome to a small-group format. *Biofeedback Self Regul.* 1987; 12(1):63-9.

4. Greene B, Blanchard EB. Cognitive therapy for irritable bowel syndrome. *J Consult Clinical Psycho l* 1994; 62(3):576-82.

5. Toner BB, Segal ZV, Emmott S, Myran D, Ali A, DiGasbarro I, et al. Cognitive-behavioral group therapy for patients with irritable bowel syndrome. *Int J Group Psychotherapy.* 1998; 48(2):215-43.

6. Van Dulmen A.M., Fennis J.F.M., Bleijenberg G. *Psychosomatic Medicine* September 1, 1996 vol. 58 no. 5.

7. Heymann-Monnikes I, Arnold R, Florin I, Herda C, Melfsen S, Monnikes H. *American Journal Gastroenterol.* 2000 Apr; 95 (4):981-94.

8. Boyce P, Gilchrist J, Talley NJ, Rose D. Cognitive-Behavior Therapy as a Treatment for Syndrome: A Pilot Study. *Aust N Z J Psychiatry.* 2000 Apr; 34 (2):300-9.

9. Boyce PM, Talley NJ, Balaam B, Koloski Na, Truman G. A Randomized Controlled Trial of Cognitive Behavior Therapy, Relaxation Training, and Routine Clinical Care for the Irritable Bowel Syndrome. *Am J Gastroenterol.* 2003 Oct; 98(10):2209-18.

10. Drossman DA, Toner BB, Whitehead WE, Diamant NE, Dalton CB, Duncan S, Emmott S, Proffitt V, Akman D, Frusciante K, Le T, Meyer K, Bradshaw B, Mikula K, Morris CB, Blackman CJ, Hu Y, Jia H, Li JZ, Koch GG, Bangdiwall SI. Cognitive-behavioral therapy versus education and desipramine versus placebo for moderate to severe functional bowel disorders. *Gastroenterology.* 2003,125: 19–31.

11. Gonsalkorale WM, Toner BB, Whorwell PJ. (2004) Cognitive change in patients undergoing hypnotherapy for irritable bowel syndrome. *J Psychosom Res* 2004 Mar; 56(3):271-8.

12. Svedlund J, Sjodin I, Ottosson JO, Dotevall G. Controlled study of psychotherapy in irritable bowel syndrome. *Lancet.* 1983; 2(8350):589-92.

13. Guthrie E, Creed F, Dawson D, Tomenson B. A controlled trial of psychological treatment for the irritable bowel syndrome. *Gastroenterology.* 1991; 100(2):450-7.

14. Creed F, Fernandes L, Guthrie E, Palmer S, Ratcliffe J, Read N, et al. The cost-effectiveness of psychotherapy and paroxetine for

severe irritable bowel syndrome. *Gastroenterology.* 2003; 124(2):303-17.

15. Blanchard EB, Greene B, Scharff L, Schwarz-McMorris SP. Relaxation training as a treatment for irritable bowel syndrome. *Biofeedback and Self Regulation.* 1993 Sep, 18(3):125-32.

16. Keefer L, Blanchard EB. The effects of Relaxation Response Meditation on the Symptoms of Irritable Bowel Syndrome: Results of a Controlled Treatment Study. *Behaviour Research Therapy.* 2001 Jul; 39 (7):801-11.

17. Kosslyn, S.M. Alpert, N.M, Thompson, W.L., Maljkovic, V., Weise, S.B., Chabris, S.F., Hamilton, S.E., and Buonanno, F.S., (1993). Visual mental imagery activates the primary visual cortex. *Journal of Cognitive Neuroscience.* 5 (3), 263-87.

Can Changes In Diet Help IBS?

1. Francis CY, Whorwell PJ. The irritable bowel syndrome. *Postgrad Med J* 1997; 73: 1–7.

2. Miller V, Lea R, Agrawal A, Whorwell PJ. (2006). Bran and irritable bowel syndrome: the primary-care perspective. *Digestive and Liver Disease* 38 (2006) 737–740.

3. Francis CY, Whorwell PJ. Bran and Irritable Bowel Syndrome: Time for Reappraisal. *Lancet* 1994 Jul 2; 344 (8914):39-40.

4. Liu JH, Chen GH, Yeh HZ, Huang CK, Poon Sk. Enteric-coated Peppermint-Oil Capsules in the Treatment of Irritable Bowel Syndrome: A perspective, Randomized Trial. *J Gastroenterol* 1997 Dec; 32(6):765-8.

Pharmacological Treatment Approaches

1. Kennedy T, Jones R, Darnley S, Seed P, Wessely S, Chalder T. Cognitive Behavior Therapy in Addition to Antispasmodic Treatment for Irritable Bowel Syndrome in Primary Care: Randomized Controlled Trial. *BMJ.* 2005 Aug 20;331 (7514):435. Epub 2005 Aug 10.

2. Drossman BA, Toner BB, Whitehead WE, et al. Cognitive behavioral therapy versus education and desipramine versus placebo for moderate to severe functional bowel disorders. *Gastroenterology* 2003; 125:19-31.

3. Tack J, Brokaert D, Fischler B, Van Oudenhove L, Gevers AM, Janssens J. A Controlled Crossover Study of the Selective Serotonin Reuptake Inhibitor Citalopram in Irritable Bowel Syndrome. *Gut.* 2006 Aug; 55(8):1095-103. Epub 2006 Jan 9.

What Have We Learned So Far?

1. Ragnarsson G, Bodemar G. Pain is temporally related to eating but not to defaecation in the irritable bowel syndrome (IBS). Patients' description of diarrhea, constipation and symptom variation during a prospective 6-week study. *Eur J Gastroenterol Hepatol.* 1998; 10(5):415-21.

2. Svedlund J, Sjodin I, Dotevall G, Gillberg R. Upper gastrointestinal and mental symptoms in the irritable bowel syndrome. *Scand J Gastroenterol.* 1985; 20(5):595-601.

3. Evans PR, Piesse C, Bak YT, Kellow JE. Fructose-sorbitol malabsorption and symptom provocation in irritable bowel syndrome: relationship to enteric hypersensitivity and dysmotility. *Scand J Gastroenterol.* 1998; 33(11):1158-63.

Is It Possible To Use Imagery In Healing

1. What Life Means to Einstein: An Interview by George Sylvester Viereck" in *The Saturday Evening Post*, Vol. 202 (26 October 1929), p. 117.

2. Papakostas YG, Daras MD. *Placebos, Placebo Effect, and the Response to the Healing Situation: The Evolution of a Concept Epilepsia.* 2001 Dec; 42 (12):1614-25.

3. Tracey I, Bingel U, Wanigasekers V, Wiech K, Mhuircheartaigh, R Ni, Lee MC, Ploner M: The Effect of Treatment Expectation on Drug Efficacy: Imaging the Analgesic Benefit of the Opioid Remifentanil. *Science Translational Medicine Journal* 16 February 2011: Vol. 3, Issue 70, p. 70.

4. Klopfer B, Psychological Variables in Human Cancer, *Journal of Prospective Techniques 31,* 1957, pp. 331-40.

5. Rossi E, W W Norton and Company, Inc., *The Psychobiology of Mind-Body Healing*, 1993.

6. Achterberg J. *Shamanism and Modern Medicine Imagery in Healing:* 2002.

7. Siebert L, Ph.D., *Naked Dreams: Hawaiian Dream Interpretation, 10 Steps To Uncovering The True Meaning of Dreams,* 2013.

8. Simonton O.C., Matthews-Simonton S., Creighton JL. *Getting Well Again*, 1978.

Can Mind-Body Communication Affect IBS Symptoms?

1. Thompson WG, Heaton KW, Smyth GT, Smyth C. Irritable bowel syndrome: the view from general practice. *Eur J Gastroenterol Hepatol* 1997; 9:689-692.

2. Lynn, S. J., Kirsch, I., Barabasz, A., Cardeña, E., and Patterson, D. Hypnosis as an empirically supported clinical intervention: The

state of the evidence and a look to the future. 2000. *International Journal of Clinical and Experimental Hypnosis,* Vol. 48, pp. 235-255.

3. Patterson, D.R., and Jensen, M.P. (2003). Hypnosis and clinical pain. *Psychological Bulletin,* Vol. 129 pp. 495-521.

4. Rainville, P., Carrier, B., Hofbauer, R. K., Bushnell, M.C., and Duncan, G.H. (1999). Dissociation of sensory and affective dimensions of pain using hypnotic modulation. *Pain,* Vol. 82, pp. 159-71.

5. Montgomery, G.H., DuHamel, K.N., and Redd, W.H. (2000). A meta-analysis of hypnotically induced analgesia: how effective is hypnosis? *International Journal of Clinical and Experimental Hypnosis,* Vol. 48, pp. 138-153.

6. Calvert EL, Houghton LA, Cooper P, Morris J, Whorwell PJ. Long-term improvement in functional dyspepsia using hypnotherapy. *Gastroenterology* 2002 Dec; 123(6):1778-85.

Summarizing The Mind Body Approach

1. Voirol MW, Hipolito J. Anthropo-analytical relaxation in irritable bowel syndrome: results 40 months later. *Schweiz Med Wochenschr.* 1987 Jul 18; 117(29):1117-9.

2. Blanchard EB, Greene B, Scharff L, Schwarz-McMorris SP. Relaxation training as a treatment for irritable bowel syndrome. *Biofeedback and Self Regulation.* 1993 Sep, 18(3):125-32.

3. Keefer L, Blanchard, EB. The effects of relaxation response meditation on the symptoms of irritable bowel syndrome: results of a controlled treatment study. *Behavioral Res Therapy.* 2001 Jul; 39(7):801-11.

4. Keefer L, Blanchard EB. A one year follow-up of relaxation response meditation as a treatment for irritable bowel syndrome. *Behavioral Res Therapy.* 2002 May; 40(5):541-6.

5. Guthrie E, Creed F, Dawson D, Tomenson B. A randomized controlled trial of psychotherapy in patients with refractory irritable bowel syndrome. *British Journal of Psychiatry.* 1993 Sep, 163:315-21.

6. Simren M, Ringstrom G, Bjornsson ES, Abrahamsson H. Treatment with hypnotherapy reduces the sensory and motor component of the gastrocolonic response in irritable bowel syndrome. *Psychosom Med.* 2004 Mar-Apr; 66(2):233-8.

7. Francis CY, Houghton LA. Use of hypnotherapy in gastrointestinal disorders. *European Journal of Gastroenterology and Hepatology.* 1996 Jun, 8(6):525-9.

8. Galovski TE, Blanchard EB. Treatment of irritable bowel syndrome with hypnotherapy. *Applied Psychophysiol Biofeedback.* 1998 Dec; 23(4):219-32.

9. Forbes A, MacAulay, S, Chiotakakou-Faliakou, E. Hypnotherapy and therapeutic audiotape: effective in previously unsuccessfully treated irritable bowel syndrome? *International Journal Colorectal Dis.* 2000 Nov: 15 (5-6):328-34.

10. Houghton LA, Calvert EL, Jackson NA, Cooper P, Whorwell PJ. Visceral sensation and emotion: a study using hypnosis. *Gut.* 2002 Nov; 51(5):701-4.

11. Barabasz A, Barabasz M. Effects of tailored and manualized hypnotic inductions for complicated irritable bowel syndrome patients. *International Journal of Clinical and Experimental Hypnosis.* 2006 Jan; 54 (1):100-12.

12. Roberts L, Wilson S, Singh S, Roalfe A. Gut-directed hypnotherapy for irritable bowel syndrome: piloting a primary

care-based randomized controlled trial. *British Journal of General Practice* 2006 Feb; 56 (523):115-21.

13. Whorwell PJ, Prior A, Faragher EB. Controlled trial of hypnotherapy in the treatment of severe refractory irritable bowel syndrome. *Lancet.* 1984 Dec 1; 2(8414):1232-4.

14. Galovski TE, Blanchard EB. The treatment of irritable bowel syndrome with hypnotherapy. *Applied Psychophysiol Biofeedback.* 1998; 23(4):219-32.

15. Forbes A, MacAulay S, Chiotakakou-Faliakou E. Hypnotherapy and therapeutic audiotape: effective in previously unsuccessfully treated irritable bowel syndrome? *International Journal Colorectal Dis.* 2000 Nov: 15(5-6):328-34.

16. Svedlund J, Sjodin I, Otosson JO, Dotevall, G. Controlled study of psychotherapy in irritable bowel syndrome. *Lancet.* 1983, Sept 10; 2(8350):589-92.

17. Svedlund, J. Functional gastrointestinal diseases. Psychotherapy is an efficient complement to drug therapy. *Lakartidningen.* 2002 Jan 17; 99(3):172-4.

18. Blanchard EB, Radnitz C., Schwarz SP, Neff DF, Gerardi MA. Psychological changes associated with self-regulatory treatments of irritable bowel syndrome. *Biofeedback Self Regulation.* 1987, Mar; 12(1):31-7.

19. Houghton LA, Heyman DJ, Whorwell PJ. Symptomatology, quality of life and economic features of irritable bowel syndrome - the effect of hypnotherapy. *Alimentary Pharmacology and Therapeutics.* 1996 Feb, 10(1):91-5.

20. Read NW. Harnessing the patient's powers of recovery: the role of the psychotherapies in the irritable bowel syndrome. *Baillieres Best Practice Res Clinical Gastroenterol.* 1999, Oct; 13(3):473-87.

21. Gonsalkorale WM, Toner BB, Whorwell PJ. Cognitive change in patients undergoing hypnotherapy for irritable bowel syndrome. *J Psychosomatic Research* 2004 Mar; 56(3):271-8.

22. Gonsalkorale WM, Houghton LA, Whorwell PJ. Hypnotherapy in Irritable Bowel Syndrome: A Large Scale Audit of a Clinical Service With Examination of Factors Influencing Responsiveness, *American Journal Gastroenterology* 2002 94 954-961.

23. Whorwell PJ, Houghton LA, Taylor EE, Maxton DG. Physiological effects of emotion: assessment via hypnosis. LANCET. 1991 Aug 15; 340(8816):434.

24. Salt WB, Neimark NF. *Irritable Bowel Syndrome and the MindBodySpirit Connection.* Parkview Publishing: Columbus, 2002.

25. Houghton LA, Calvert EL, Jackson NA, Cooper P, Whorwell PJ. Visceral sensation and emotion: a study using hypnosis. *Gut.* 2002 Nov; 51(5):701-4.

Why Use Gut-Directed Hypnosis For The Treatment Of IBS?

1. Whorwell PJ, Prior A, Faragher EB. Controlled trial of hypnotherapy in the treatment of severe refractory irritable-bowel syndrome. *Lancet.* 1984; 2 (8414):1232-4.

2. Whorwell PJ, Prior A, Colgan SM. Hypnotherapy in severe irritable bowel syndrome: further experience. *Gut,* 1987; April, 28(4):423-5.

3. Harvey RF, Hinton RA, Gunary RM, Barry RE. Individual and group hypnotherapy in treatment of refractory irritable bowel syndrome. *Lancet.* 1989 Feb; 1(8635):424-5.

4. Houghton LA, Heyman DJ, Whorwell PJ. Symptomotololgy, quality of life and economic features of irritable bowel syndrome –

the effects of hypnotherapy. *Alimentary Pharmacological Therapy.* 1996, Feb, 10(1):91-5.

5. Palsson, O.S., Burnett, C.K., Meyer, K., and Whitehead, W.E. (1997). Hypnosis treatment for irritable bowel syndrome. Effects on symptoms, pain threshold and muscle tone. *Gastroenterology,* 112, A803.

6. Palsson, O.S., Turner, M.J., Johnson, D.A., Burnett, C.K., and Whitehead, W.E. (2002). Hypnosis treatment of severe irritable bowel syndrome: Investigation of mechanism and effects on symptoms. *Digestive Diseases and Sciences,* 47(11): 2605-2614.

7. Galovski TE, Blanchard EB. The treatment of irritable bowel syndrome with hypnotherapy. *Applied Psychophysiol Biofeedback.* 1998; 23(4):219-32.

8. Palsson OS, Turner MJ, Johnson DA, Burnett CK, Whitehead WE. Hypnosis treatment for severe irritable bowel syndrome: investigation of mechanism and effects on symptoms. *Dig Dis Science* 2002 Nov; 47(11):2605-14.

9. Gonsalkorale WM, Houghton LA, Whorwell PJ. Hypnotherapy in irritable bowel syndrome: a large-scale audit of a clinical service with examination of factors influencing responsiveness. *American Journal of Gastroenterol.* 2002 Apr, 97(4):954-61.

10. Gonsalkorale WM, Miller V, Afzal A, Whorwell PJ. Long term benefits of hypnotherapy for irritable bowel syndrome. *Gut.* 2003 Nov; 52(11):1623-9.

11. Galovski TE, Blanchard EB. Hypnotherapy and refractory irritable bowel syndrome: a single case study. *American Journal of Clinical Hypnotherapy* 2002 Jul; 45(1):31-7.

12. Houghtom LA, Calvert EL, Jackson NA, Cooper P, Whorwell PJ. Visceral sensation and emotion: a study using hypnosis. *Gut* 2002 Nov; 51(5):701-4.

13. Gonsalkorale WM, Toner BB, and Whorwell PJ. Cognitive change in patients undergoing hypnotherapy for irritable bowel syndrome. *Journal of Psychosomatic Research* Volume 56, Issue 3, March 2004, Pages 271–278.

14. Bennett EJ, Piessea C, Palmer K, Badcock C-A, Tennant CC, Kellow JE. Functional gastrointestinal disorders: psychological, social, and somatic features. *Gut* 1998; 42 pages 414-420.

15. Wilson S, Maddison T, Roberts L, Greenfield S, and Singh S; Systematic review: the effectiveness of hypnotherapy in the management of irritable bowel syndrome. *Aliment Pharmacol Therapy.* 2006 Sep 1; 24(5):769-80.

What is the Typical Protocol for Gut-Directed Hypnotherapy?

1. Gonsalkorale, W.M., Houghton, L.A., and Whorwell, P.J. (2002). Hypnotherapy in irritable bowel syndrome: a large-scale audit of a clinical service with examination of factors influencing responsiveness. *The American Journal of Gastroenterology*, 97 (4), 954-961.

2. Whorwell, P.J., (2006). Effective management of irritable bowel syndrome - the Manchester model. *International Journal of Clinical and Experimental Hynposis*, 54 (1), 21-26.

3. Galovski, T.E. and Blanchard, E.B. (2002). Hypnotherapy and refractory irritable bowel syndrome: a single case study. *American Journal of Clinical Hypnosis*, 45 (1), 31-37.

4. Zimmerman, J. (2003). Cleaning up the river: a metaphor for functional digestive disorders. *American Journal of Clinical Hypnosis*, 45 (4), 353-359.

5. Kraft, T. and Kraft, D. (2007). Irritable Bowel Syndrome: symptomatic treatment approaches versus integrative psychotherapy. *Contemporary Hypnosis,* 24 (4), 161-177.

6. Gonsalkorale, W.M. Gut-directed hypnotherapy: the Manchester approach for treatment of irritable bowel syndrome. *International Journal of Clinical and Experimental Hypnosis,* 2006. 54 (1), 27-50.

7. Kearney, D.J., and Brown-Chang, J., Complementary and alternative medicine for IBS in adults: mind-body interventions. *Nature Clinical Practice Gastroenterology and Hepatology,* 2008. 5, 624-636.

Conclusions

1. Brandt LJ, Chey WD, Foxx-Orenstein AE, Schiller LR, Schoenfeld PS, Spiegel BM, et al. An evidence-based position statement on the management of irritable bowel syndrome. *American Journal Gastroenterol.* 2009; 104 Suppl 1:S1-35.

2. Mykletun A, Jacka F, Williams L, Pasco J, Henry M, Nicholson GC, et al. Prevalence of mood and anxiety disorder in self reported irritable bowel syndrome (IBS). An epidemiological population based study of women. *BMC Gastroenterolol.* 2010; 10(1): 88

www.ingramcontent.com/pod-product-compliance
Lightning Source LLC
Chambersburg PA
CBHW060617290526
45793CB00001B/64